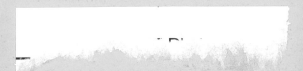

OXFORD MEDICAL PUBLICATIONS

Manual on Methodology
for Food Consumption
Studies

MANUAL ON METHODOLOGY FOR FOOD CONSUMPTION STUDIES

MARGARET E. CAMERON

and

WIJA A. VAN STAVEREN
(editors for IUNS and EURO-NUT)

OXFORD UNIVERSITY PRESS
1988

Oxford University Press, Walton Street, Oxford OX2 6DP

Oxford New York Toronto
Delhi Bombay Calcutta Madras Karachi
Petaling Jaya Singapore Hong Kong Tokyo
Nairobi Dar es Salaam Cape Town
Melbourne Auckland

and associated companies in
Berlin Ibadan

Oxford is a trade mark of Oxford University Press

Published in the United States
by Oxford University Press, New York

British Library Cataloguing in Publication Data
Manual on methodology for food consumption
studies.
1. Food. Consumption. Assessment. Manuals
I. Cameron, Margaret, 1921–
II. Staveren, Wija A. van
339.4'86413
ISBN 0–19–261577–7

Library of Congress Cataloging in Publication Data
Manual on methodology for food consumption studies/[edited by]
Margaret E. Cameron and Wija A. van Staveren; editors for IUNS and
EURO-NUT.
Bibliography:
Includes index.
1. Nutrition surveys—Methodology—Handbooks, manuals, etc.
2. Nutrition—Research—Methodology—Handbooks, manuals, etc.
I. Cameron, Margaret, 1921–   . II. Staveren, Wija A. van.
III. International Union of Nutritional Sciences.   IV. EURO-NUT.
TX367.M35   1988   363.8'2'028—dc19   88-5189
ISBN 0–19–261577–7

Typeset by Cotswold Typesetting Ltd, Cheltenham
Printed in Great Britain
at the University Printing House, Oxford
by David Stanford
Printer to the University

FOREWORD

Professor Mahmoud K. Gabr, President IUNS, Cairo, Egypt
Professor Joseph G. A. J. Hautvast, Project Leader EURO-NUT,
Wageningen, The Netherlands

The science of human nutrition is coming of age. More and more people with interests in basic biomedical sciences, internal medicine, dietetics, epidemiology, and public policy at the national and international level are studying the relationship between man and his food. Much of this work is directed towards:

- identification of people consuming various foods and determining the quantities of such foods consumed;
- characterization of dietary patterns of a population in relation to social, cultural, economic, and health status;
- determination of the quality of food in relation to nutritional requirements; and
- examination of the relationship of nutrient intake with health, well-being, and disease.

One of the most difficult, time-consuming, and therefore expensive components of research directed towards these aims is the measurement of food intake either in individuals or in groups of persons ranging from few in number to millions. For a variety of reasons not only do people differ in their food intake but also one person can consume quite different foods and amounts of food on various days, in various months or in various years. Although we are aware that such variations do exist, it is necessary to have precise information on the regular dietary intake both at the level of the individual and of the group. Over the last few decades, careful attention has been given by nutrition scientists to the development of adequate methods for the measurement of dietary intake. However, it is surprising that the methods which are reported in scientific papers are poorly designed and inadequately described. Thus, it is often impossible to compare the results of different studies and, as a consequence, progress in nutrition science is slowed down. Therefore, it can be concluded that there is a great need for basic information on how dietary intake should be measured in various types of studies under a variety of conditions.

For many years, the International Union of Nutritional Sciences (IUNS) has been active in this field of work through a working group charged with the responsibility of developing a manual of techniques for the measurement of dietary intake. The working group had close contact with another working group with somewhat similar aims which was established within the framework of EURO-NUT which is the Concerted Action Programme on Diet and Health of the Commission of the European Communities.

As representatives of IUNS and EURO-NUT, we have great pleasure in presenting to you the fruit of the co-operation between the two working groups, now ready for harvest. The fruit is in the form of the new *Manual on methodology for food consumption studies*. We consider that this book is unique because no comparable book on this subject has been written for 25 years. It will be invaluable during the planning and execution of research and in teaching students techniques for the measurement of food intake.

Many nutritional scientists with a wide range and depth of experience have been involved in writing this book. To them, we express our sincere thanks for imparting their knowledge and for their perseverance in completing their task. In particular, we would like to thank the editors of the manual, Miss Margaret Cameron and Dr Wija van Staveren, for their work over a number of years on this project. They were responsible for guiding this work to completion through discussions with the authors of the various chapters to whom they gave constant support. We feel that the community of nutrition scientists will be grateful for many years to come for the preparation of this manual.

ACKNOWLEDGEMENTS

We would like to acknowledge with thanks the financial support of EURO-NUT and IUNS for the preparation of this manual. In particular we owe thanks to Professor Dr J. G. A. J. Hautvast who, much earlier, was present when the idea for such a manual was born and has given us constant encouragement and good advice.

Apart from the main contributors who responded so well to our many requests, and mostly on time, it would be difficult to name everybody who has helped us in our task. But we would like to thank the members of the working group who formed the final editorial committee, Sheila Bingham and Johanna Haraldsdottir. Our thanks go also to Jan Burema who so generously gave valuable advice and constructive criticism on chapters other than his own; to Riet Hoogkamer who most cheerfully and carefully typed the manuscript; and to Jean H. Sabry who, with one of us (W. A. van Staveren) helped to write the original manual outline, five years ago.

We also acknowledge authors and publishers, who have given the permission to include certain figures and photographs.

CONTENTS

4   Purposes of food consumption studies   25

5   Methods for data collection at household or institutional level   33

10 Validity and reproducibility 171

11 Validation problems 183

12 Obtaining food consumption data in special circumstances: additional considerations

14 **Practical implementation**

EDITORS

Margaret Cameron has a degree in Home Science from New Zealand and postgraduate dietetic training. Before becoming principal lecturer in Nutrition and Dietetics at the Polytechnic of North London she worked with the late Professor Platt in the Department of Human Nutrition at the London School of Hygiene and Tropical Medicine. Latterly she has been an honorary senior lecturer to the Tropical Child Health Unit, Institute of Child Health, University of London.

She has had the experience of teaching students from all over the world, conducting training courses and consultancies for WHO and other agencies.

Wija van Staveren worked as a research dietitian at the Central Institute for Food and Nutrition Research TNO, Zeist, (The Netherlands) before she joined the Department of Human Nutrition of the Wageningen Agricultural University in 1972. In 1973 and 1974, she had the opportunity to study for the degree of Master of Science in Human Nutrition at Queen Elizabeth College of the University of London and in 1985, she obtained a Ph.D. degree from the Wageningen Agricultural University based on her research on the validity and reproducibility of food intake measurements. She is senior lecturer in Human Nutrition in Wageningen where she participates in teaching in the university's degree course as well as in international education programmes. Her research involves measurement of food consumption in populations in the Netherlands, in Europe and in developing countries.

CONTRIBUTORS

Lenore Arab, M.Sc., Ph.D., Department of Epidemiology of Health Risks, Institute for Social Medicine and Epidemiology, Federal Health Office, Berlin, FRG.

Sheila A. Bingham, Ph.D., Dunn Nutrition Unit, University of Cambridge and Medical Research Council, Cambridge, United Kingdom.

Alison E. Black, B.Sc., SRD, Dunn Nutrition Unit, University of Cambridge and Medical Research Council, Cambridge, United Kingdom.

Piet A. van den Brandt, M.Sc., Department of Epidemiology, University of Limburg, Maastricht, The Netherlands.

Jan Burema, Statistician, Department of Human Nutrition, Agricultural University, Wageningen, The Netherlands.

Margaret E. Cameron, B.H.Sc., SRD, Nutritionist. Present address: 42 Highgate, Roslyn, Dunedin, New Zealand.

Elizabeth Campbell Asselbergs, M.Sc., Formerly Nutrition Officer Food Policy and Nutrition Division FAO, Rome. Presently: 95 Westgate Park Drive, St. Catharines, Ontario, Canada L2N 5X1.

Marina Flores, Instituto de Nutricion de Centro America y Panama, Guatemala, Central America.

Jean H. Hankin, Professor of Public Health and Research Nutritionist, University of Hawaii at Manoa.

Johanna Haraldsdottir, M.Sc., Department of Nutrition, National Food Agency, Copenhagen, Denmark.

Wijnand Klaver, M.Sc., International Courses in Food Science and Nutrition, Wageningen, The Netherlands.

Jan T. Knuiman, Ph.D., Department of Human Nutrition, Agricultural University, Wageningen, The Netherlands.

Elin Bjørge Løken, M.Sc., Section for Dietary Research, Institute for Nutrition Research, Faculty of Medicine, University of Oslo, Norway.

Michael Nelson, M.Sc., Ph.D., Department of Food and Nutritional Sciences, King's College London, University of London, United Kingdom.

Alison A. Paul, B.Sc., Dunn Nutrition Unit, University of Cambridge and Medical Research Council, Cambridge, United Kingdom.

Ingrid H. E. Rutishauser, B.Sc. (Nutrition), Division of Biological Sciences, Deakin University, Geelong, Victoria, Australia.

Jean Henderson Sabry, Ph.D., Professor of Applied Human Nutrition, Department of Family Studies, University of Guelph, Guelph, Ontario, Canada N1G 2W1.

David A. T. Southgate, Ph.D., MI Biol., Agricultural and Food Research Council, Institute of Food Research, Norwich Laboratory, Norwich, United Kingdom.

Wija A. van Staveren, Ph.D., RD, Department of Human Nutrition, Agricultural University, Wageningen, The Netherlands.

TABLES

FIGURES

1

A historical look at manuals for food consumption studies

Review of the original two manuals on dietary surveys published by FAO in 1949 and 1962

MARINA FLORES

In 1945, during the first Food and Agricultural Organization (FAO) conference in Quebec, Canada, it was pointed out that one of the tasks of the new international organization should be the preparation of a booklet on the methodology used for dietary surveys. FAO had stressed repeatedly the importance of household food consumption surveys, which supplemented food balance sheet data and provided information over and above that of the balance sheets. The nutritionist, Thelma Norris, was assigned by the Nutrition Division of FAO to complete the task and in 1949 she published an excellent report, *Dietary surveys: their technique and interpretation.* It was designed to 'assist workers undertaking dietary studies in different parts of the world'.

The great value of this report was the extensive bibliography which was compiled and classified, subject by subject, by Thelma Norris. Practically all the dietary surveys carried out before 1948 were analysed and described in the report. However, because few surveys had been carried out in developing countries, and in some none at all, the only available studies which could be included came from Western Europe and North America. Most of these had been carried out in urban areas. This meant that the techniques and methods described were appropriate only for those countries whose social and economic structures and dietary habits were similar in character.

The reports of the first classic dietary surveys, conducted by the pioneers in this field, provided the scientific basis of the Norris report. Among those presented were the experiences of Isabella Leitch, Great Britain; E. J. Bigwood, Belgium; Hazel Stiebling, United States of America; F. W. Clements, Australia; and J. Trémoliere, France.

There are descriptions of the main steps taken to plan and organize the surveys along with the methods used to implement them. The terminology differs from more recent publications, but essentially it has the same meaning. Four types of unit were surveyed: the total population of a country; homogeneous groups; families; and individuals.

With regard to methodology, Norris described the inventory (or log book) and the food list methods for family surveys. For homogeneous groups, which include institutional studies, two methods were mentioned. One referred to the weighing of all food as it entered the central kitchen and the weighing of all refuse and waste. The second, for experimental purposes, studied each individual; all food portions served were weighed and each item used in any composite food mixture recorded. Norris also described the dietary history of individuals using questionnaires, precise weighing methods, and chemically analysed aliquots.

Her report included a set of rules to follow when drawing the statistical sample for a survey, to ensure that the size would include all major variations in the dietary patterns of the group being studied. Good guidelines for the selection and training of field personnel were also given.

A section of great value described the combined studies of families and individuals, and aimed to show how food was distributed among different family members. This description was based mainly on the experiences of Leitch, who had used this combined method to obtain more precise information. Finally, one chapter was devoted to studies in developing areas, describing their possible objectives and organization. The information was derived from the studies of A. G. van Veen (in the Far East), J. M. Bengoa (in Venezuela), and R. K. Anderson (in the Mezquital Valley of Mexico). A good description of the two methods used to collect data, including the weighing of meals, was given along with the details of other information considered necessary, especially if it concerned food preparation and the recipes used.

The second document, *Manual on household food consumption surveys, 1962*, was prepared by Emma Reh, also an FAO nutritionist, and differed from the earlier publication. FAO had recognized that more direct methods of study were needed if information was to be obtained about the food consumption of largely illiterate food-producing rural communities. To study such groups dietary survey teams would have to visit each household and record, by weighing, the quantities of all foods eaten during a specific period.

Reh's manual is concerned with these types of dietary survey, dealing both with the collection of food consumption data and their interpretation in terms of nutrient value and in relation to nutritional requirements as they were then known.

Surveys were to be made, not only to discover what people ate but also to find information which would provide a basis for improving their dietary practices. The success of education in nutrition was recognized as being dependent on the knowledge and understanding of the many factors which influence food consumption. This comprehensive manual described, in great detail, the steps to be followed when conducting household food consumption surveys, especially in rural communities. The reason for the practical excellence of the manual is that each statement resulted from the extensive experience of Reh, herself, who carried out many surveys in different regions of the world, but especially in Latin America.

Nutritionists involved in food consumption studies, following the instructions that she described, will immediately realize that many problems were anticipated during the stage of planning and organizing a survey. All the steps to be considered in the organization of the fieldwork are well described in logical order. In addition, the instructions are presented in such a way that the manual is most enjoyable to read as well as being a rich source of information for teachers and students of nutrition.

Reh stressed the importance of the preliminary visit to the survey area, when the purpose is to obtain general information on socio-economic facts and the environmental setting. Such information is essential for good planning of a field study. The human aspects of surveys are extensively discussed, not only in relation to the population to be surveyed but also to the fieldworkers. Guidelines for the selection and training of the survey team are provided along with suggested aspects of the social sciences which should be part of any study.

For those who are not specialists in mathematics, a chapter is devoted to statistical techniques that can be used to select the representative sample to be surveyed.

Great emphasis was given to all aspects considered necessary for obtaining information about the characteristics of different members of the food consumption group, which in nearly all human societies is the family. Thus the many ways of studying the family sources of food, of obtaining food weights, monetary values, and of dealing with foods coming from the family crops are given.

Another section discusses the art of describing foods; a very important aspect for survey records because of the many factors which change or influence chemical composition and therefore nutritional values. Reh recognized that even if a food had the same name, its nutrient value depended on its freshness, whether it was raw or cooked, dried or salted, pickled or smoked. Flours from cereals and other seeds could be refined to different degrees with changed nutrient values. Thus the edible or net weights of foods must be calculated from their gross or purchased weight by using different conversion or wastage factors. The manual presents all the possibilities regarding these weights, for vegetables and fruits, foods from animal origin, and the percentage of extraction of grains.

In 1947, FAO recommended uniform and improved methods with

which to calculate a food's calorific and nutrient value, the purpose being to help revise protein, carbohydrate, fat, and energy values given in older food composition tables. This was an important step in attempting to calculate as accurately as possible the nutrient value of foods, especially those which were eaten in large quantities. These calculations could be used to show the contribution made to total diet by the various food groups in terms of nutrients and the proportion of total calories which came from protein, carbohydrate, and fat. The collected food consumption data, interpreted into calorie and nutrient values could then be related, per head, per day, to the published nutrient requirements, according to the age, sex, and activity of the population being investigated.

Calories and nutrients could also be shown in terms of their relative cost or monetary value. The contribution of the different food groups could be costed in the same way. Reh included the appropriate tables with specific physiological factors to be applied to individual foods when calculating calorie values from protein, carbohydrate, or fat.

Food consumption surveys require specialized procedures, often requiring much effort and expenditure, but Reh thought that it might be desirable to combine them with, for example, multi-purpose surveys and gave guidelines for proceeding in this direction. Other aspects which might be included were health, economics, and agriculture, as they all relate to food consumption, housing, farming, income, and family expenditure as well as all the possible economic resources of the family. They could all be used in a more comprehensive nutritional assessment throughout the country. Given in an appendix, the forms used to gather information are interesting to read. They include forms to collect: a type of census within the survey community to find out family composition details of sex, age, civil status, educational levels, occupations, and physical details of height and weight; socio-economic data relating to household facilities, use, tenancy, and size of land holdings or number of animals; family income and type of employment and family expenditure. There were special forms to record daily food consumption in the household and a summary of these; a record form for gross weights, monetary values, and origins of foods; a form to record those present at each meal in the survey period along with their age and sex; and, finally, a schedule to record the analysis of the foods consumed.

The most important limitation of this interesting manual for the present day, is that it includes only one method of dietary survey—weighing and recording—which is very precise. There was no discussion of other possibilities to modify or adapt the method for other kinds of studies, which must be done with different purposes in mind. Nevertheless, in its time this manual has been a classic.

The reasons for preparing the present manual will become obvious when the next chapter has been read.

References

Norris, T. (1949). *Dietary surveys: their technique and interpretation.* Food and Agricultural Organization of the United Nations, Rome.

Reh, E. (1962). *Manual on household food consumption studies.* Food and Agricultural Organization of the United Nations, Rome.

2

Purpose, content, and limitations of the manual

MARGARET E. CAMERON

Introduction

Along with the historical background of food consumption studies, Chapter 1 has discussed Emma Reh's manual, published by FAO for international use. At that time many studies were being carried out to determine how much food was being consumed by families and other groups, most of them in households in the developing world.

Since 1962, the reasons and circumstances for studying food consumption have changed considerably. Though time and money may still be scarce resources, opportunities for training personnel have improved at all levels. A wider range of suitable equipment and related resources for field use can be obtained. Better facilities and techniques for laboratory analyses of foods and biochemical materials have been developed. New technology provides computers, including data banks and data processing facilities. More use can be made of epidemiological studies and there is increased appreciation of the necessity to have a sound statistical basis in the design of any project. The reasons for studying food consumption to make dietary assessments has widened considerably. Methodologies have been designed to meet these needs which vary from sophisticated research studies to simple 24-hour dietary recalls. Cross sectional, longitudinal, retrospective, and prospective studies investigating individuals or groups, in precise or more general terms, are now being carried out in many places. Studies have become more detailed and specialized. For all these reasons, it became clear that there was a need to update and extend the first international manual. That is the intention of this manual. It is, however, no longer feasible to expect one person to be an expert in all aspects of food consumption studies. For this reason different authors, writing on the basis of their own experience and expertise, have contributed to the writing of this text.

7

2.1. The purpose of an international manual on food consumption methodology

The main purpose is to meet the new developments in this field. There is a variety of reasons for making such studies and there are different methods one can use to make measurements and collect data. Furthermore, there is a need to improve the analyses of data and presentation of results.

It is intended that this manual should be a reference for international use. It should, therefore:

(1) enable international studies to be planned more efficiently and effectively;

(2) ensure that comparisons made between countries are valid;

(3) provide the means for clearer communication and better understanding on all aspects of food consumption studies;

(4) share information and experience relating to new methodologies.

2.2. The manual content

The manual content has been arranged to progress logically from the first stage of deciding on the study's purpose, through its design, to collection of data, analyses, interpretation, and, finally, to the presentation of results in a form suitable for the specific study and any decision making.

The terms used throughout this manual are defined in Chapter 3. The correct use of terms should lead to greater survey accuracy, more clarity in expressing results, and greater confidence that valid comparisons could be made between one study and another. Correct use of terms would also provide a good basis for effective communication between all personnel planning and implementing surveys.

Because food consumption studies are done for different reasons, Chapter 4 discusses a variety of possible purposes so that the aim of the study which is to be undertaken can be defined with clarity.

Chapters 5 and 6 are concerned with methodology. They discuss the principles, practical aspects, advantages, disadvantages, and limitations, as well as the validity of the different methods used to collect different types of information on food consumption of individuals or groups of subjects. The basic components in methods assessing food consumption are:

● the way of collecting data, for instance by record or recall;
● the estimation of the amounts of foods eaten; and
● the conversion of foods into nutrients.

Chapter 7 discusses the technical aspects which are important for the efficiency of data collecting.

Chapter 8 discusses the use of direct analyses of foods and the setting up and use of food composition tables and nutrient databases both for national and international use.

Analyses of collecting data, their interpretation, and the presentation of results has many potential pitfalls. How to anticipate these in practice and to reduce them to a minimum is explained in Chapter 9.

Chapters 10 and 11 deal with validity, reliability, or reproducibility and accuracy. In Chapter 10, concepts are explained, guidelines to validate a selected method are given, and, for reproducibility, the need for a knowledge of variability is explained. Chapter 11 looks at what has happened in practice by surveying published studies and using firsthand experience. It attempts to set, in a practical context, the problems that have occurred, in the hope that the validity of results in future might be accepted with more confidence.

Chapter 12 proposes certain modifications in methodology which are sometimes necessary to meet special circumstances of, perhaps, human disabilities or geographical difficulties. For these a different approach for data collection might be needed.

Human and material resources always seem to be in short-supply when carrying out food consumption studies. Chapter 13 gives an economic appraisal of various study designs and methods in terms of personnel, equipment, transport, accommodation, and computing.

Finally, Chapter 14 has undertaken the important task of using the information and advice from all the other chapters and along with practical experience, shows how it can be implemented in practice. In a step-by-step approach, a study is defined, planned, and taken to the stage where its results must be presented in such a way as to suit its purpose. The examples, figures, and tables given are a useful addition to this chapter.

2.3. Using the manual

In any reputable text with tables of food composition, the reader is first requested to read the introduction. It is hoped that readers will follow the same advice before using this manual.

Each chapter is a complete account of its own specific topic, though it might be supported and extended by others which precede or follow it. Each is broken down into sections and shows the names of those who contributed to it. It also has a list of references. However, throughout the manual, to avoid unnecessary repetition and to emphasize the relationships between chapters, cross references have been made. A maximum of three figures has been used to do this. Thus, (3.1.1.) would be a cross reference to Chapter 3, section 1 and subsection 1. This would take the reader back from a later chapter to a definition given earlier. Tables and figures are indexed in a similar way. Fig. 8.1, for example, would be the first figure to be found in Chapter 8.

Literature references used for each topic are numbered and listed in alphabetical order at the end of the chapter. In the manual text, to make reading easier, each reference(s) is indicated by its number at the relevant place. Reference 6 would be listed as the sixth reference at the end of its chapter. If more than one reference is mentioned at one time the numbers would be separated by commas. For example references 6, 10 would be listed as the sixth and the tenth references at the end of the appropriate chapter.

2.4. Limitations of the manual

Of necessity the manual has a general approach. No manual written for international use would be able to cover the specific needs of every geographical region around the world. Nor could it meet all of the many purposes for which food consumption data may be needed. Nor is it feasible to give specific examples to illustrate all situations.

Where possible, some examples have been given to emphasize, qualify, or illustrate points that have been made. However, in spite of this limitation, it is intended that the guidelines and information given in this manual will help in the selection of the most appropriate method for the study to be done.

Where adjustments or modifications are made at any stage in the methodology and for whatever reason, then their possible effects should be assessed by referring to the critical discussions given on methods and techniques.

In some situations investigators are interested in the intake of only one or two specific nutrients. Considering such specific purposes for some nutrients, e.g. sodium and potassium, the preferred method of assessing intake might be by use of a biological marker (sodium and potassium in 24-hour collections of urine). Though biological markers are occasionally mentioned in a few chapters, it was considered beyond the scope of this manual to describe the particular technique in any detail.

This manual on methodology for food consumption studies will be useful in most situations, particularly for collaborative studies. It should help to make planning more efficient and effective, and it should ensure that valid comparisons can be made with confidence.

3

Definitions of terms

WIJNAND KLAVER, JAN BUREMA,
WIJA A. VAN STAVEREN, AND JAN T. KNUIMAN

Introduction

In the introduction to this manual it is stated that the use of well-defined terms would prevent confusion and enhance the value of published results from food consumption studies. This chapter emphasizes the statement by providing the preferred definitions for the terms used.

In 1982, a EURO-NUT workshop on *Methods of evaluating nutritional status with emphasis on food consumption*[6] proposed definitions for use in the methodology for such studies. With minor amendments those definitions are presented here in four sections.

Section 3.1. considers basic concepts at various levels: food supply; food consumption; and food utilization. These concepts are summarized in Fig. 3.1. Terms on patterns of food consumption and types of surveys are summarized in Fig. 3.2.

Section 3.2. gives definitions of measuring techniques, by type. There are, however, other ways to classify techniques. Examples of these are:

(1) by level—individual/household/region;
(2) by directness—direct/indirect, including accounting/recording/recalling.

Section 3.3. is concerned with the techniques assessing food consumption and using direct analysis for the conversion of data into energy and nutrients.

Section 3.4. deals with basic statistical concepts and includes terms for correctness of measurement. These terms are summarized in Fig. 3.3.

In this chapter it should be noted that where reference is made to an author, the text given in the publication cited will not necessarily be in the form of a definition. In the literature, it is very difficult to find definitions which are concerned with the various aspects of food consumption studies.

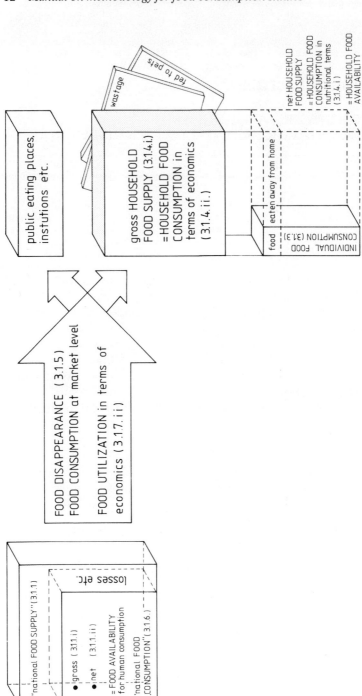

Fig. 3.1. Basic concepts of food supply, consumption, and utilization.

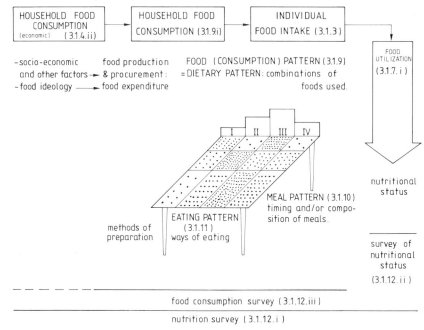

Fig. 3.2. Basic concepts of food patterns, consumption, and types of surveys.

3.1. Definitions for basic concepts

3.1.1. Food supply

Gross food supply is the sum of production and procurement (purchase, barter, receipt, or imports) of foods, minus sales, exports, and decreases in stocks.

Net food supply is the gross food supply minus losses in transport and storage and minus non-human uses of food (e.g. feed, seed, manufacture of non-consumable products).

In food balance sheets (3.2.2), the net food supply is worked out at retail level. If a further deduction is made for losses at household level, one obtains a figure that can be used as a more or less indirect measure of the total quantity of foods available per capita, for food consumption.

Synonym: food availability.

3.1.2. Food consumption

This is the food and drink ingested. In the first stage it is expressed by type of food or drink. The measurement can be in terms of quantities or of frequencies of the different types of food or drink ingested during a given time unit per individual or household. In a later stage of analysis, foods and drinks may be grouped together, provided the common denominator is appropriate for the purpose of the analysis.

In general it is not appropriate to add the weight of different foods without correction for their different water contents. The ultimate expression of quantities consumed is in terms of energy and nutrients (3.3).

Synonyms: food intake; dietary intake.

3.1.3. *Individual food consumption*

This is the food and drink ingested by an individual.

3.1.4. *Household food consumption*

Household food consumption in a nutritional sense represents the food and beverages consumed by the household.

This can be the sum of the food intakes of the individual household members, or it can be the total amount of food consumed in the household, excluding that eaten away from home unless taken from home. The user of this term should specify which alternative has been used.

Household (food) consumption in an economic sense is the sum of the (food) commodities purchased, or obtained by other means, by the household.

It is expressed in terms of food 'as purchased'. It includes the amounts of food purchased for pets, and the loss or wastage of food such as trimmings, spoilage, or plate waste. In budget surveys, food is one of the elements of household 'consumption'.

3.1.5. *Food disappearance*

This refers to the 'disappearance' of food commodities through all existing distribution channels (i.e. by the various categories of users, such as households, public eating places, and institutions).

Synonyms: food consumption at market level; food utilization (in the economic sense).

3.1.6. *National food consumption*

This is assessed by a food consumption survey performed on a representative national sample. (N.B. Food balance sheet data (3.2.2) should not be referred to as 'food consumption', but rather as 'food supply' or 'food availability'.)

3.1.7. Food utilization

Food utilization in terms of physiology is the process whereby nutrients are absorbed and metabolized by the organism.

Food utilization in terms of food economics, is the quantitative breakdown into various categories of use of real or potential food supply.[5]
Synonym: food use.

3.1.8. Food-related patterns
A pattern is a repeated arrangement of components into combinations, as observed. A pattern is not a reality, it is instead a way of looking at reality. A pattern often arises when data are being analysed. The rationale behind 'patterning food consumption within time periods'[3] is that the patterns may vary from group-to-group and from situation-to-situation. As such, patterns are considered to be intervening variables between socio-economic and psycho-cultural factors of food behaviour on one hand and intake of nutrients by the individual on the other.

3.1.9. Food patterns
These are repeated arrangements that can be observed when foods are eaten. This refers particularly to the type and relative proportions, and/or the combinations of foods used in meals by an individual, a given community, or population group. These combinations can be expressed quantitatively in various ways, e.g. weight, nutrient content, or money value of the foods.
Synonyms: food consumption patterns; dietary patterns.

3.1.10. Meal patterns
Meal patterns can be defined in two ways: in terms of food consumption patterns according to meals, as the repeated arrangements that can be observed for the distribution of foods most frequently consumed by individuals, their relative proportion and approximate amounts according to the various meals of the day; or in terms of patterns of mealtimes, as repeated arrangements that can be observed in the usual number of meals per day and the times at which they are served.

3.1.11. Eating patterns
This term is used in a variety of ways to describe combinations of foods eaten together; variations in times and places of eating; social functions of meals (including eating companions); and variations in food consumption of households or individuals. There is no consensus on a single meaning of the term.

3.1.12. Surveys
Nutrition survey is a survey which aims to collect information about the nutritional status and dietary intake of a population group or category.

Survey of nutritional status is a survey of population groups in order to determine their state of nutrition by clinical, biochemical, and/or anthropometrical measurements.

Food consumption survey is a survey designed to obtain qualitative and/or quantitative information on the food actually eaten.

A comprehensive food consumption survey should include in addition, the collection of information on socio-economic and other factors relevant to food consumption.[5]

Synonym: dietary survey.

3.2. Definitions for measurement techniques

There are indirect and direct methods for the assessment of food consumption. Accounting techniques measure everything but food consumption itself and are thus an indirect method (3.2.2–3.2.4). Food consumption can be assessed directly by recording techniques (3.2.5–3.2.11) or by interview techniques (3.2.12). (N.B. In social sciences the terms technique and method do not have the same meaning. In this manual, however, the terms will be used as synonyms.)

Synonym: method.

3.2.1. Accounting techniques

3.2.2. Food balance sheet

This is a national account of the annual production of food, changes in food stocks, imports and exports, and distribution of food for various uses within the country. It thus provides an indirect estimate of the *per capita* supplies available for human consumption. This account can be prepared on the basis of the calendar year, the agricultural year, or the crop year. The various uses are listed under the following headings: animal feed; seed; industrial uses; waste; and the net food availability for human consumption at the retail level. *Per capita* food availability is given for the total population actually partaking of the food supplies during the reference period, i.e. the population present within the geographical boundaries of the country at the mid-point of the reference period. In some countries, the *per capita* food availability refers only to the civilian population, the armed forces being excluded. *Per capita* food availability is expressed in grams of food and in amounts of energy and of some nutrients.

In the various countries, national food accounts may be called 'foods moving into consumption', 'food disappearance data' or 'food consumption statistics'; the accounting techniques used may differ also.

3.2.3. Food account method (household)

A method that uses a record of all food purchases and food brought into the household from other sources during a 7-day period or longer. This measure assumes that there have been no significant changes in household food reserves over the period of the study.[2] The optimal number of days to be observed per household, depends on the variation in food and shopping habits.

3.2.4. Inventory method (household)

A method that uses a record of all purchases (cf. food account method) *and* changes in food reserves of the household generally over a period of a week. At the beginning and end of this period an inventory is made of all food in the house. All foods brought into the house during this period are also recorded.[2]

3.2.5. Recording techniques

The term 'recording' refers to the record of current food intake. Observation is made during the consumption period, in contrast to other techniques of direct assessment, which are based on retrospective recall. The unit of observation may be the household (3.2.6) or the individual (3.2.7–3.2.11). Amounts of foods may be weighed or weights can be estimated with the help of household measures, food models, and/or photographs (7.1.2–7.1.5). Associated energy and nutrient content can be obtained from food composition tables. If foods need to be analysed other techniques are applied (3.3).

In this manual a household measure is the volume associated with known household utensils or with usual portion sizes. Utensils include cups, spoons, tins, and so on.

3.2.6. Household record method

This aims to weigh or estimate, in household measures, the (raw) foods available for consumption in the household on a particular day. This is sometimes done during daily visits by fieldworkers. Foods not eaten by the household members should be subtracted.

3.2.7. Precise weighing record

A record kept by the subject of the weights of all ingredients used in the preparation of the meals, as well as the inedible waste, the total cooked weight of meal items, the cooked weight of the individual's portion, and plate waste. (N.B. The word 'precise' in this context refers to the complete coverage of the measurements, i.e. food is weighed also before preparation, rather than to the precision of the scale measurements.)

3.2.8. Weighed record

A record of foods weighed by the subject immediately before consumption and of all plate waste, edible and inedible, weighed at the end of the meal. Standard recipes may or may not be used. (If the ingredients are weighed before preparation then we call the method precise weighing record.)

Synonym: weighed inventory record.

3.2.9. Estimated record

A record kept by the subject of all foods eaten using various ways to estimate the weight of the foods, for example household measures, food models, or photographs. In the description of the method the various ways should be specified.

3.2.10. Observed weighed (estimated) record

The record kept by a fieldworker instead of the subject, is called an 'observed weighed record' when foods are weighed immediately before consumption. In the 'observed precise weighing record' the ingredients used in the preparation of meals are also weighed. When the weights of foods are estimated with the help of household measures, food models, or photographs, the method is called 'observed estimated record'.

3.2.11. Menu record

This is a record kept by the subject with descriptions of the kind of foods eaten, but without any attempt to quantify the amounts.

3.2.12. Interview techniques/methods

Interview methods use an interviewer and are based on a recall of foods consumed by the respondents. As with the recording technique, the unit of observation can be the household or the individual (3.2.6, 3.2.7–3.2.11). Amounts of foods already eaten cannot be weighed on scales, therefore the weights of foods are estimated using household measures, food models, or photographs. In the description of the method the way the amount of food was estimated should be specified.

3.2.13. List–recall method

Used at household level, this is a procedure in which the interviewer lists major food items in a structured questionnaire to help the respondent to recall the amount and price, or purchase value, of all foods used in the household in a specified period, often 7 days.

3.2.14. 24-hour recall method

Used at individual level, is a procedure to find out, by means of an interview, the actual food intake of an individual during the immediate past, usually 24 or 48 hours, or the preceding day. Food quantities are usually assessed by using household measures, food models, or photographs.

Synonym: daily recall method.

3.2.15. Dietary history method

This is a procedure where the interviewer assesses an individual's total usual food intake and meal pattern. During interviews, the respondent is asked to provide information about his/her pattern of eating over an extended period of time and also to recall the actual foods eaten during the preceding 24 hours. In addition, the interviewer completes a checklist of foods usually consumed. Finally as a cross-check, the respondent is asked to complete a 3-day esimated record.

Considerable confusion exists in the literature on the details of a 'dietary history method'. Several modifications have been used. Furthermore, the term 'cross-check method' is *not* recommended as a synonym for 'dietary history method' as the cross-check method is only a part of the dietary history method. Furthermore, the cross-check can also be used as part of a recall method.

3.2.16. Food frequency method

A procedure which estimates how often foods are eaten by an individual. The frequency is usually qualitative and is expressed per day, week, or month. The food frequency method may include quantitative assessment of usual portion sizes.

3.3. Conversion of food consumption data into energy and nutrients by direct analysis

The energy and nutrient composition of the foods eaten can be estimated from food composition tables or by direct analysis. In the following methods, the intake of nutrients by the individual is assessed by means of direct analysis of a food sample which is directly comparable to the food consumed by the individual.

3.3.1. Duplicate portion technique

A technique in which equivalent portions of all foods and beverages consumed by an individual, are collected for direct analysis in order to estimate the individual's intake of energy, nutrients, and/or other food constituents. Often equivalent portions of water are omitted from the collection. The samples may be combined or separated.

3.3.2. Aliquot sampling technique

A technique in which all foods and beverages consumed by an individual during the survey period are weighed. Aliquot samples (i.e. a specified proportion of all foods and beverages, with or without water) are collected daily. Subsequently, the composition of the aliquot samples, taken during the whole survey period are estimated by direct analysis. The samples may be combined or separated.

3.3.3. Equivalent composite technique

A technique in which the weights of all foods and beverages consumed by an individual (often water is omitted) are recorded during the whole survey period. Afterwards a combined sample of raw foods, equivalent to the mean daily amounts of food eaten by an individual during the survey period, is directly analysed.

3.4. Definitions for basic statistical concepts

Definitions of terms relating to the accuracy of measurements are given in this section. There are various sources of error and variation in the estimation of food consumption (Fig. 3.3). These sources of error and variation influence the quality of the ultimate result of the study.

Sources of error and variation	Terminology	
Systematic imperfectness of information	Validity	Accuracy
Systematic response error		
Random response error	Reproducibility (precision)	
Biological within-person variation		
Biological between-person variation	Representativeness	
Misinterpretation by selection of sample and/or by selection of days		

Fig. 3.3. Sources of error and variation in the estimation of food consumption.

3.4.1. Systematic errors *versus* random errors

The terminology used to qualify a method of measurement reflects the two kinds of error that play a part in every investigation, namely systematic and random errors.

A *systematic error* is the tendency of a measurement to produce on average, an over- or under-estimation of what the method is intended to measure. Such a systematic error causes a bias in the estimation. As an example, if, in a dietary history, a respondent tends to consistently over-estimate the amounts of food of his/her weekly consumption, the estimated energy intake will be biased.

Random error: whether the method under consideration is biased (has systematic error) or not, a particular assessment of someone's food intake on a particular day may differ from his actual consumption that day for various reasons, e.g. errors in the estimated amounts of foods consumed, foods omitted, or coding errors. These errors, as far as they are not systematic, are called random errors. On average they may cancel out, but they affect the precision of the estimated mean intake.

3.4.2. Validity

Validity is an expression of the degree to which a measurement measures what it purports to. Consequently, any systematic error of the measuring instrument affects the validity of the measurement. The validity of a method to estimate food consumption should be assessed by comparing its results with those of another method of indisputable quality. However, no method exists that is known to be absolutely free from bias, because of the nature of food consumption data of free-living individuals. Therefore, it is common to choose a food consumption method of general acceptance, as the reference method. It can then be said that the 'relative validity' of a method with respect to another method has been assessed. Two examples follow:

1. A 24-hour recall method is tested against the results of the observed and preferably weighed amounts of food eaten during the same period. Thus, a synonym of relative validity is comparative validity. If the results of a food consumption method are validated against some external criterion, it is also called the comparative validity.

2. The 24-hour protein intake as estimated from a record or recall method may be evaluated against the nitrogen excretion in a 24-hour urinary sample from the same person in the same period.

N.B. In practice the term validity is often used without adding 'absolute', 'relative', or 'comparative'.

3.4.3. Reproducibility

The reproducibility of a method is the extent to which it produces the same results, when applied repeatedly in the same situation. The smaller the within-person variability the better the reproducibility.

However, it should be emphasized that for any measure of variability, it is very important to specify what is meant by 'the same situation'. When someone's habitual intake is the object of the study, day-to-day variability in current (actual) intake is a source of variation that contributes to the imprecision of the measurement.

As an example, the reproducibility of a dietary history method, when habitual intake is being assessed, is better then the reproducibility of a 2-day record method, because of day-to-day variability. However, the latter may be improved by taking records over 4 or 5 days.

In addition, seasonal variations may or may not be included in the reproducibility. Thus, when a dietary history is taken from the same subject on two occasions 3 months apart, a seasonal variation may contribute to the imprecision when information on food consumption during the previous 3 months is being considered. However, the assessment of someone's yearly habitual dietary intake may be more reproducible.

Synonyms for reproducibility are: repeatability, reliability, replicability, precision.

3.4.4. Accuracy

In this manual the term accuracy is connected with validity and reproducibility. Both systematic and random errors detract from the accuracy of the measurement.

3.4.5. Representativeness of the subjects under study

This is the extent to which the distribution of relevant variables in sample and target populations are the same. For metabolic experiments, under controlled conditions, these variables are restricted to physiological variables. In observational studies with free-living populations in addition to physiological variables, situational variables have to be considered.

3.4.6. Representativeness of the period of observation

This is important in studies on free-living individuals. Representativeness, in this context, is the extent to which the distribution of relevant variables is the same in both the period of observation and the time-frame in which the investigator wants to generalize the results of the study.

Bibliography

1. Block, G. (1982). A review of validation of dietary assessment methods. *Am. J. Epidemiol.* **115**, 492–505.

2. Burk, M. C. and Pao, E. M. (1976). Methodology for large-scale surveys of household and individual diets. *Home Economics Research Report No. 40.* USDA. Washington D.C.
3. Burk, M. C. and Pao, E. M. (1980). Analysis of food consumption survey data for developing countries. *FAO Food and Nutrition Paper No. 16.* FAO, Rome.
4. Burke, B. S. (1947). The dietary history as a tool in research. *J. Am. Diet. Ass.* **23**, 1041–6.
5. FAO/WHO. (1974). Food and nutrition terminology. *Terminol. Bull. No. 28.* FAO, Rome. (N.B. This document does not constitute formal publication).
6. Klaver, W., Knuiman, J. T. and van Staveren, W. A. (1982). Proposed definitions for use in the methodology of food consumption studies. In *EURO-NUT Report 1,* (Hautvast, J. G. A. J. and Klaver, W., eds) pp. 75–85, Wageningen.
7. Last, J. M. (1982). Towards a dictionary of epidemiological terms. *Intl. J. Epidemiol.* **11**, 188–9.
8. Marr, J. W. (1971). Individual dietary survey: purpose and methods. *World Rev. Nutr. Diet.* **13**, 105–64.
9. Worsley, T. (1981). Psychometric aspects of language dependent techniques in dietary assessment. *Trans. Menzies Found.* **III**, 161–94.

4

Purposes of food consumption studies

JEAN HENDERSON SABRY

Introduction

Food consumption data are collected for a variety of purposes. The most relevant to this manual are purposes related to: food and nutrition planning; nutritional studies; and toxicological aspects of the food supply. Some examples are given in this chapter.

Before commencing any food consumption study or survey, it is important to define the purpose. Both the design of the study and the method selected for measuring food consumption depend upon the purpose for which data will be used. Methods for collection of food consumption data and their uses are described in Chapters 5 and 6.

The planning of a study must include considerations of statistical design, sampling, and statistical treatment of data. Participation of statisticians from the early stages is essential to avoid later problems in statistical analysis and interpretation of results. (Chapters 9 and 14.)

The availability of suitable food composition data is important when the consumption of energy, nutrients, and other food constituents is being investigated. Many regional and national tables of food consumption are available in printed and computer-retrievable forms. Considerable differences exist among these tables.[6] In addition, data are lacking on the nutrient content of many foods and for many nutrients.[8] International cooperation in the generation and interchange of reliable food composition data is promoted by the International Network of Food Data Systems (INFOODS).[7] The completeness of available food composition data with respect to the needs of each particular study must be considered. Decisions must be made on the handling of missing food composition values, for example, whether to substitute with compositional values for a similar food, to use values calculated from recipes and ingredient lists, or to obtain missing values by laboratory analysis. Particular attention should be given to those foods comprising the core diet of the population and to the specific nutrients of interest. The use of food composition tables is discussed in 8.2.

4.1. Purposes associated with national food and nutrition planning

4.1.1. Adequacy of the food supply

Food and nutrition planning requires information on the quantities of food available and the adequacy of the food supply to meet the needs of the population. National data, such as food balance sheets or food disappearance are usually reported annually. From these data, the *per capita* amounts of energy, protein, and other nutrients in the national food supply can be calculated. These *per capita* data describe the food availability, but not food consumption. Food and nutrient losses prior to consumption, due to processing, spoilage, trimming, waste, and cooking, may not be adequately accounted for. Furthermore, *per capita* data make no allowance for the uneven distribution among different population groups and different geographic regions, or for seasonal differences. *Per capita* data are useful in that they give an indication of the adequacy or inadequacy of the available food supply. Data on the *per capita* available food supply can be described in terms of composition by food group, for example, by amounts of cereals, pulses, milk, meat etc., and in terms of nutrient composition, that is, by levels of energy, protein, fat, carbohydrate, and vitamins and minerals. Where food supplies are marginal or inadequate, *per capita* data provide direction for planning food production, for regulating food imports and exports, and setting priorities for food aid. Where food supplies are ample, data on macro-nutrients and micronutrient levels of the food supply can help to identify changes that would be considered desirable in terms of health. National data are especially useful for assessing trends over time in the *per capita* energy and nutrient levels of the food supply and may help in the formulation of hypotheses for studies on the relation of diet to health. Methods for the collection of food availability at the national level are considered to be outside the scope of this manual.

4.1.2. Food production and food distribution

Food and nutrition planning is concerned with setting targets for food production to increase an inadequate food supply, with developing programmes to improve the nutritional quality of the food supply, and with assessment of changes in food production, food imports, and food exports from year-to-year. Data for these purposes are obtained from food balance sheets.

Information as to how the available food supply is distributed among different segments of the population is important in the identification of target groups for social programmes. Information on food distribution is obtained by studies of food consumption at the household or individual level. These studies do not assess channels of food distribution directly. Rather, they measure the end result of food distribution (Fig. 3.1) as indicated by differences in food consumption among populations in different geographic areas and in different income groups.

4.1.3. Food regulations, food fortification, and nutrition education

Development of food regulations, including regulations on food fortifications, and of food guides for use in nutrition education programs requires information on food consumption patterns and on the contribution of a specific food or food group to the intake of nutrients. Data on food consumption collected at the household and individual level contribute to the description of the food consumption patterns of the population as a whole and of various population groups.

4.2. Purposes with a nutritional focus

4.2.1. Estimation of the adequacy of dietary intakes of population groups

Studies to estimate the adequacy of dietary intake require the collection of food consumption data at the individual level of assessment. It is important for the design of a study to clarify whether the purpose is to assess the adequacy of the average intake of a group or to determine the proportion of individuals within the group having adequate or inadequate intakes. In the latter case the method selected for collection of food consumption data must provide information on the average intake of the group and on the distribution of the group intake as discussed in Chapter 6.

Classification of the adequacy of intakes is made by comparison with a reference value, usually one based on recommended intakes or allowances. Where recommendations formulated within a country are available, they are commonly used as the reference. For other countries the nutrient requirements published by FAO/WHO may be used.[4, 10] Recommended intakes of protein, minerals, and vitamins, however, are customarily set above the average requirement to cover the needs of almost all healthy people in the population. For many nutrients the recommended intake represents the average requirement plus two standard deviations, on the assumption that individual requirements are normally distributed.[3, 9] Since the recommended intake is greater than the requirement of nearly all persons in the population, the prevalence of inadequacy is overestimated if the recommended level is used as the criterion of dietary adequacy. For this reason it has been customary to use cut-off points, often set at two-thirds or three-quarters of the recommended intake, to estimate the proportion of a population with inadequate intakes.

It has been pointed out that the classification of nutrient intakes on the basis of recommended intakes, or cut-off points based on them, is likely to lead to errors in the estimation of the prevalence of inadequacy.[1] To avoid this limitation, a probability approach to the estimation of nutrient adequacy has been proposed.[3] The probability approach takes into account both the distribution of nutrient intakes in the population and the variability of nutrient requirements. The probability approach cannot be applied to energy intakes or nutrients for which information about the variation in requirement among individuals is lacking. Application of the probability approach to the interpretation of nutrient intake data is discussed in Chapter 9.

In theory, the probability approach is applicable to the estimation of risk for excessive nutrient intake. However, for most nutrients there is insufficient information to define the level at which intakes become excessive and the variability of that level.

Classification of nutrient adequacy on the basis of nutrient intake data alone provides only a relative estimate since nutrient intake measures are insufficient to describe nutritional status. In surveys where biochemical, anthropometric, and clinical measures of nutritional status are obtained, dietary data should be interpreted in conjunction with these biological measures to determine the proportion of populations at risk for inadequate or excessive intakes of nutrients.

4.2.2. Investigation of relationships of diet to health and nutritional status

Many nutrition studies are undertaken to investigate relationships of diet to nutritional status and the role of diet in the development of chronic diseases. There are numerous examples of relationships between a dietary factor and a measure of health or nutritional status. Some examples are: salt intake and blood pressure; type and quantity of dietary fat and serum cholesterol; amount and frequency of consumption of sugar and the number of decayed, missing, or filled teeth; type and amount of dietary fibre and colonic function; protein intake and calcium excretion; vegetarian diet patterns and iron status. In most cases, investigation of such relationships requires collection of data on the individual's usual or habitual diet. The reader is referred to Chapter 6 for a discussion of possible methods.

The choice of method for the collection of food consumption data and the design of each study will vary greatly depending on the nature of the relationship being examined, the specific dietary characteristic(s) under investigation, and the time period of interest for food consumption, i.e., current diet, usual diet, or past diet. Design considerations would include appropriate sampling, whether to sample randomly selected populations groups, groups with unusual food consumption patterns (for example high salt consumption), or groups with a specific physiological characteristic, such as hypercholesterolaemia. It is important in the design and statistical analysis to control for possible confounding effects from other dietary factors and health or nutritional conditions upon the relationship under investigation (Chapter 8).

4.2.3. Evaluation of nutrition education, nutrition intervention, and food fortification programmes

Measures of food consumption can play an important role in the evaluation of nutrition programmes. Where the aim of community nutrition education programmes and food fortification programmes is to reduce the number of persons within a group having inadequate or imbalanced nutrient intake, considerations in the assessment of food consumption are similar to those described above for estimation of adequacy of nutrient intakes. Frequently nutrition education programmes are undertaken to bring about specific change in food choices in line with nutrition guidelines for good health. Evaluation of such programmes might include pre- and post-programme measures of frequency of consumption of a restricted list of appropriate foods, to obtain group data.

Nutrition intervention programmes are aimed at lowering risk factors and disease in a target group. In some programmes food consumption is an outcome variable, i.e., a measure of programme effect. In other studies food consumption is a mediating variable, i.e., an influence on the effectiveness of the programme. An example is seen in intervention programmes providing supplementary food items to individuals or households. To evaluate the impact of a supplementary food programme on health status, it would be important to find out the extent to which the supplementary food items increased food and nutrient intake, replaced foods from other sources, or were not consumed by the target population. In clinical nutrition intervention trials, food consumption may act as a measure of adherence to a modified eating pattern and as a mediating variable influencing an outcome measure, such as body weight or serum cholesterol.

When the purpose of the study is to compare the response of an intervention group with a control group, it may be sufficient to collect food consumption data which provides group averages. If the survey design requires correlational or multivariate analysis of the food consumption variable, a method for individual diets should be used.

4.3. Purposes associated with toxicological aspects of the food supply

4.3.1. Estimation of average intakes of food additives and contaminants

Information on the intake of food additives and food contaminants such as heavy metals and pesticide residues is needed to determine whether or not they constitute a health risk. Intakes of these compounds may be estimated from food consumption data which describe the relative contribution of individual food items or food groups to the diet. The level of additives or contaminants in the diet can be calculated if levels of the compound in food items and food groups are known or have been obtained by direct analysis. An alternative approach, called a total diet study, involves direct analysis of a composite diet, or of food group composites, formulated in proportion to average consumption patterns.[2, 5] Estimation of the average consumption of additives or contaminants by different population groups requires collection of food consumption data at the individual level. This data would also provide information about maximum and minimum levels of intake. The average consumption of the population as a whole can be estimated by weighting of the food consumption data on population groups. Data from national household food consumption surveys may also be used to provide estimates of average levels of additives and contaminants in the national diet.[2]

4.3.2. Estimation of habitual high and low levels of consumption of foods containing fortification nutrients and food additives

In order to define safe levels of fortification nutrients and additives in foods, it is necessary to consider not only the average amount of the substance consumed, but habitual high levels of intake. Additionally, in fortification programmes it is helpful to know what proportion of the population is not likely to benefit due to habitually low intake levels of the foods which have been fortified. This information can be obtained, for different population groups, from household or individual surveys of food consumption, provided the data permit estimation of the distribution of usual food intake in the group. When information is needed on patterns of intake of certain specific food items, it may be more efficient to use a quantitative food frequency questionnaire (6.8).

References

1. Beaton, G. H. (1986). Toward harmonization of dietary, biochemical, and clinical assessments: The meanings of nutritional status and requirements. *Nutr. Rev.* **44**, 349–58.
2. Ministry of Agriculture Fisheries and Food. (1978). *The surveillance of food contaminants in the United Kingdom.* Food Surveillance Paper No. 1. HMSO, London.
3. National Research Council (1986). Nutrient Adequacy. *Assessment using food consumption surveys.* Food and Nutrition Board, Subcommittee on Criteria for Dietary Evaluation, Washington.
4. Passmore, R., Nicol, B. M., Rao, M. N., Beaton, G. H. and Demayer, E. M. (1974). *Handbook on human requirements.* WHO Monograph Series No. 61, Geneva.
5. Pennington, J. A. T. (1983). Revision of the total diet study; food lists and diets. *J. Am. Diet Assoc.* **82**, 166–73.
6. Périssé, J. (1982). The homogeneity of food composition tables. In: *The diet factor in epidemiological research* (Hautvast, J. G. A. J. and Klaver, W., eds) pp. 100–5. Wageningen.
7. Rand, W. M. and Young, V. R. (1984). Report of a planning conference concerning an international network of food data systems (INFOODS). *Am. J. Clin. Nutr.* **39**, 144–51.
8. Stewart, K. K. (1983). The state of food composition data. *Food Nutr. Bull.* **5(2)**, 54–68.
9. Truswell, A. S. (1983). Recommended dietary intakes — introduction. In: Recommended dietary intakes around the world. A report by the Committee 1/5 of the International Union of Nutritional Sciences (1982). *Nutr. Abstr. Rev.* **53**, 939–46.
10. WHO (1985). *Energy and protein requirements.* WHO Technical Report Series No. 724.

5

Methods for data collection at household or institutional level

MARINA FLORES AND MICHAEL NELSON

Introduction

Several outstanding studies on methodology to evaluate food consumption at household or institutional level have been published during the last 40 years.[2, 6, 16, 17, 20, 22] The abundance of the literature in this field is due mainly to the diversity of food behaviour and food patterns among the cultural and socio-economic population groups of different countries. Each specific society demands a methodology which is adjusted to the economic and environmental factors affecting the families living there.

In this chapter the four methods most commonly used to estimate either the gross or the net household food supply will be described (Fig. 3.1). The purpose of the study will determine which type of information is needed (Chapter 4):

(1) for economic purposes, the *gross* household food supply and the amount of money spent on it should be determined;

(2) for nutritional purposes, the *net* household food supply or availability of nutrients should be estimated.

Common characteristics of methods to assess household food availability are:

1. The unit of observation. This will be a household, family group, or institution. It is necessary to have a complete description of the members who participate in eating the daily meals of the unit, with records of their individual age, sex, occupation or activity level, and physiological state.

2. Quantities of foods purchased and eaten. This can be based on the number and weight of retail units purchased, foods described in household measures or comparable food models, or the prices of foods purchased where price per unit weight is known (7.1.2–5). The most accurate information, of course, is obtained by actually weighing the foods (7.1.1).

3. The optimal number of days to observe per household, and the

optimal number of households in the study. This depends on the variation in food and shopping habits within and between households, and the level of accuracy required for estimates of either food consumption of nutrient intake.

5.1. Principles of the methods

5.1.1. Food account method (3.2.3)

When applying the food account method for family surveys, the housewife* or fieldworker must keep a day-by-day record of the amounts of all foods purchased for the family during the period of the study. Foods obtained as gifts or payments in kind and home produced foods must be included in this record.

This method assumes either that there are no significant changes in the food reserves or stores within a household during the study, or that when the results are averaged over a sufficient number of households (e.g. 20) that the net gains and losses in larder stocks in the individual households will cancel each other out. For an estimate of nutrients available to household members, it is necessary to make an allowance for waste and for food consumed by visitors. Foods eaten outside the home will also contribute to total nutrient intake, but may not be included in the reported figures for consumption.

An example of this method is found in the *Household food consumption and expenditure survey of Great Britain.* It is carried out each year amongst a nationally representative sample of approximately 7,500 households.[15] In this study, the housewife records for 7 days the weight (and, if possible, the price) of all food entering the household for human consumption.

5.1.2. Inventory method (3.2.4)

In this method, a fieldworker takes an inventory of all food in the household at both the beginning and the end of the survey period. The fieldworker or housewife also records the weights of all foods brought into the house during this same period. Thus, the only difference between this and the food account method is that changes in the food reserves or stores of individual households are taken into account. This method was used in Great Britain before 1951 for a number of surveys including *The urban working-class household diet, 1940–49.*[16] Although it gives a more accurate estimate of nutrient intake than the food account method, it

*Synonyms: housekeeper, housemother, person (male or female) in charge of meal preparation or domestic duties.

distorts normal food purchasing patterns by drawing respondents' attention to existing larder stocks[12,13] and therefore has limited value for economic purposes.

5.1.3. Household record method (3.2.6)

This method may be used when information is wanted on the foods available for consumption in the household during the day(s) of observation. The amounts of food prepared and served may be weighed or estimated in household measures* by the housewife or fieldworker. Foods eaten other than by household members should be weighed or estimated and the amount subtracted from the total amount available for consumption.

Subjects in the survey may individually record foods obtained and eaten outside the household (14.2.1). When the amounts of all the foods eaten are totalled, it should give a complete account of the food consumption for all subjects during the study period.

This method has been used in a study of the food habits of 90 Guatemalan Indian families[7] and, in a modified form, in a study of the energy balance of army recruits.[4]

5.1.4. List–recall method (3.2.13)

In this method, the interviewer uses a list of major food items in a structured questionnaire to help the respondent recall the amount and price of all foods used in the household during the period of study. It is similar to the food account method, but it estimates food used as well as food purchased and it requires only a single interview as it is based on recall rather than a current record. The method is used in the United States National Household Food Consumption Surveys[24] and has been analysed in detail.[2]

5.2. Practical aspects in household surveys

The approach to household surveys will depend on:

(1) whether food brought into the house is mainly purchased or home produced;

(2) how food is prepared;

(3) whether a direct estimate of the net amount of food available for consumption is required, or if an indirect estimate based on adjusted gross figures is sufficient;

*See 3.2.5.

(4) the degree of literacy of the respondent;

(5) the number of interviewers available;

(6) the time period to be studied.

5.2.1. Food account and inventory methods

The recording of data in the food account and inventory methods has been described in 5.1.1. It involves simple record keeping of the gross amounts of food available for human consumption within the household. A diary is kept of the foods served at meals during the study period in order to check that foods served were also recorded as having entered the house and that foods with a short shelf-life were actually consumed. In order to know how many household members ate the food and how many of their meals were obtained from outside the household food supply, it is also necessary to record the age and sex of subjects present at each meal, including any visitors. Examples of forms for recording such data are shown in Figs 5.1. and 5.2.

5.2.2. List–recall method

The list–recall method is also straightforward in principle. Care must be taken to compile a comprehensive list of foods likely to be consumed in the study population. If the housewife is given advance warning of the study in a letter, she may be able to keep receipts and make notes of foods purchased or coming into the household which will assist her during the recall. This will improve the accuracy of the data recalled, but may have the disadvantage of drawing attention to the survey and altering normal purchasing patterns. It is important to determine the amount of food *used* as well as the amount brought into the household, as the food usage data will improve the accuracy of the estimate of net food consumption within the household. As in the food account method, it is necessary to obtain a list of the age and sex of people eating meals from the household food supply during the period of the study.

5.2.3. Household record method

The procedure for the household record method is more complex. It involves a mixture of recall and recording. The following outline is based upon recommendations of the Institute of Nutrition of Central America.[14]

At the first home visit the fieldworker should:

(1) give a simple explanation of the study to the housewife;

(2) inquire about the best hour(s) of the day for subsequent visits;

FOOD COMING INTO HOME

FOOD BOUGHT AT NORMAL PRICES .... DAY [**-1**]

Oz, lbs, pints, or number	Grammes, kilos or litres	DESCRIPTION OF FOOD *Please describe ITEM in full and give BRAND* *Use one line for each ITEM*	COST £	COST p.	PLEASE LEAVE BLANK Food	PLEASE LEAVE BLANK Q
						1
						1
						1
						1
						1
						1
						1
						1
						1
						1
						1
						1
						1
						1
						1
						1
						1
						1
						1
						1
						1
						1
						1
						1
						1
						1

HOME GROWN FOOD, GIFTS, FREE MILK, SCHOOL MILK, WELFARE FOOD

Oz, lbs, pints, or number	Grammes, kilos or litres	DESCRIPTION OF FOOD	SOURCE Garden, farm, school, clinic, employer, own business, etc	FREE OR COST £	FREE OR COST p.	PLEASE LEAVE BLANK Food	PLEASE LEAVE BLANK Q	PLEASE LEAVE BLANK Free

FOR OFFICE USE

340			343			346			349		
341			344			347			350		
342			345			348					

6

Fig. 5.1. Example of form to record weights, descriptions, and costs of food entering the household.

MEALS

	1 BREAKFAST	2 MID-DAY MEAL	3 TEA OR AFTERNOON MEAL	4 EVENING MEAL OR SUPPER
What did you serve?				
How many of the people on the front of this book ate the meal at home?	Number of people	Number of people	Number of people	Number of people ....

Did you have any visitors for this meal? FEMALE = F MALE = M	VISITORS TO BREAKFAST		VISITORS TO MID-DAY MEAL		VISITORS TO TEA		VISITORS TO EVENING MEAL	
	SEX	AGE	SEX	AGE	SEX	AGE	SEX	AGE

Did anyone obtain a meal out? (for which you did not provide the food). Where was it eaten? FEMALE = F MALE = M	BREAKFAST OUT			MID-DAY MEAL OUT			TEA OUT			EVENING MEAL OUT		
	SEX	AGE	WHERE?	SEX	AGE	WHERE?	SEX	AGE	WHERE?	SEX	AGE	WHERE?

Did anyone take a packed meal from home to eat out? FEMALE = F MALE = M	PACKED BREAKFAST		PACKED MID-DAY MEAL		PACKED TEA		PACKED EVENING MEAL	
	SEX	AGE	SEX	AGE	SEX	AGE	SEX	AGE

Contents of a packed meal? Who did not have a meal? FEMALE = F MALE = M				

15

Fig. 5.2. Example of form to record meals served in the household and details of who ate them. (Courtesy, National Food Survey Branch, Ministry of Agriculture Fisheries and Food, UK.)

(3) make a register of the household members' age, sex, occupation or activity level, and physiological state;

(4) record the time and a description of that day's breakfast. This includes estimated amounts of foods, beverages, and ingredients of the items served, and, also, who was present at the meal.

(5) list the time and description of the next meal, obtaining the weights of raw ingredients to be used; include any bread, cakes, fruit, or beverages to be consumed. The food weights, if possible, should be of the edible portions which will have been prepared and are ready for cooking or to be eaten raw.

If the study period is only one day, the second visit should be on the afternoon of the same day and:

(1) ask again about lunch for cross-checking purposes;

(2) list the weights and the kinds of foods to be used for the evening meal;

(3) record who was present at lunch and ask who will attend the evening meal.

If the study period is more than one day, the second visit could be made the next morning. The information about the previous evening meal and this day's breakfast will be obtained by the recall method (6.5). The amounts of food will be estimates. The weights of foods to be used for the following meal will then be recorded.

The description of each food item should include details of its kind, variety, and quality;

(1) whether it is fresh, canned, dried, salted, pickled, or fermented and the name of any brand;

(2) for meats, the kind and part of the animal;

(3) for cheese, the type of milk used to make it and whether it is hard, semi-soft, or soft;

(4) for the staple grain, whether whole grain or refined flour is used.

It is essential to be aware of all conditions which might change the nutritive value of food. It is important to make a note of cooking methods, especially for the staple food. For example, the use of lime water to soften maize increases its calcium content and liberates nicotinic acid which is otherwise bound in niacytin.

An account should be taken of food wasted or given to animals. Food may be wasted at three points; between coming into the house and preparation, between preparation and serving, and after serving (plate waste). Where it is not possible to measure waste directly, an estimate should be made in order not to overstate the quantity of food and nutrients available. Respondents probably reduce the amount of waste when it is being measured directly.

The success of the interview and the accuracy of the information obtained depends on the personality and training of the fieldworker (7.2.3).

5.3. Practical aspects in institutional surveys

Central catering in institutions provides an opportunity to obtain records of food prepared for consumption by large numbers of individuals. From these records estimates of the average nutrients available per person can be calculated. Such surveys require the full cooperation of the institution's catering staff. As in household surveys, a list is required giving the age and sex of subjects being catered for and the number of meals consumed.

Data collection in institutions can be carried out using the inventory method or the household record method, provided they are modified appropriately.

The inventory method in institutions depends upon an accurate record of the total amount of raw materials purchased for catering. Estimates of food consumption and nutrient intake should allow for losses in storage, preparation, and cooking. Plate waste may be estimated by collecting and weighing all uneaten food and allocating to each food an amount of waste in proportion to the weight of food served.

The household record method in an institution depends upon a knowledge of standard portion sizes. This can be determined either by actually weighing out representative portions of foods, or by calculation from recipes which give the weights of raw ingredients to be used per 100 portions (or other fixed number). Allowances for cooking losses (e.g. evaporation water) must be made when calculating portion size. From a record of the total number of portions of each food served and the standard portion sizes, the total amount of food available for consumption can be calculated. The sex and age of those eating the food during the survey period must also be recorded. An example of this type of dietary survey is reported in a study of diet based on 7000 menu cards completed by hospital in-patients on 10 wards in a large general hospital in Portsmouth, England.[26]

If the diet of subjects is not provided wholly within the institution, then a record of the number and type of meals eaten outside should be obtained. It may also be necessary to estimate amounts of food being given to subjects which comes from outside the institution's food supply (gifts of food from visitors to patients in a hospital, for example). Plate waste should be estimated.

5.4. Uses and limitations

Household survey methods provide a quick way of estimating the food consumption and nutrient intake of communities, be they villages, towns, or institutions. With appropriate sampling and care in interpretation (5.6), comparisons can be made between communities, regions, income groups, household types, and other socio-economic categories.

The food account and inventory methods are particularly suitable for record keeping by respondents in communities where foods are mainly purchased and the level of literacy is high. They can also be used effectively where the interviewer has frequent access to the larder or stores and can obtain, by recall, the amounts of foods withdrawn from stocks for meals. They are especially useful for estimating gross food supply and providing economic data.

The household record method is of value in providing direct estimates of the net amount of food available, especially in surveys in which interviewers make regular visits to the respondents. It is better suited than the food account method to communities in which a substantial proportion of food is home produced and the level of literacy is low.

The list–recall method can also be used to make net estimates of food available, but is dependent on a recall of the weights of foods over a longer time period. It has the advantage of requiring only a single interview, but is subject to the disadvantages of any survey which is based on memory.

5.4.1. Period of study

The majority of household surveys cover a period of one week. This is the period in which the pattern of acquiring household food is likely to repeat itself. Shorter periods may be used provided a bias is not introduced. There is some evidence to show that a one week recording period using either the food account or list–recall methods may result in an overestimation of actual consumption (5.6). This problem may be overcome by recording diet for a longer period, as the tendency to 'stock up' in the first week is unlikely to continue into a second week. Both the inventory and household record methods overcome this problem by assessing the amount of food actually consumed (allowing for visitors, pets, and waste), but data on purchasing is then biased and the pattern of consumption may not be normal.

It is essential to be aware of the effect of seasonality on the availability of foods. This may be especially important when comparing two apparently similar communities using data from surveys conducted at different times of the year. There may also be some advantages in conducting studies over an entire year in order to obtain a complete picture of food availability.

5.4.2. Interviewer and respondent burden

One of the main advantages of household surveys is the relatively large amount of information which is obtained for comparatively little effort. The most efficient procedure is the list–recall because a single interview is sufficient to obtain the information required. The next most efficient procedure is the food account method. This usually requires three visits from the interviewer. It places a great burden upon the respondent, who must keep a record of all food acquisitions for the survey period. Greater effort still is needed from both the interviewer and respondent in the inventory method, as it requires all the work associated with the food accounts method plus very lengthy interviews at the beginning and end of the study period to complete the inventories. A shift of the burden from the respondent to the interviewer is achieved in the household record method, which makes it more appropriate in studies where the level of literacy in the population is low.

In institutional surveys, the 'respondent' may in fact be the catering officer rather than the study subject. Care must be taken to allocate sufficient research sources to an institutional survey. While the catering officer may be able to provide access to the desired information, it is unlikely that he/she will have time to collect the data needed. It may therefore be necessary for the interviewer to spend several weeks (or months) abstracting the data from catering records.

5.4.3. Limitations

There are a number of important limitations to household surveys, such as:

1. They record food availability, not consumption. Food which is wasted, or given to visitors or pets may be incorrectly included in the estimate.

2. Food obtained from outside the household food supply is not recorded. Unless each household member keeps a record of food obtained from outside the household food supply, the results will relate only to a part of the diet.

3. Certain foods may not be recorded. In the National Food Survey of Great Britain, for example, sweets, soft drinks, and alcoholic beverages are not recorded even if purchased for home consumption. This avoids the distortion which would occur when comparing families which consume these items either mainly at home or mainly away from home.

4. Purchasing patterns may be distorted. In the food account method, Nelson *et al.*[20] have shown that average purchases are 15 per cent in excess of measured home food consumption. It has also been shown that normal patterns of purchasing are altered as a result of the larder survey in the inventory method, though this may only occur where larder stocks are extensive and highly varied.[13] Memory may distort the true pattern of purchases in the list–recall method.

5. No information on the distribution of foods within households or institutions is normally obtained. If this information is needed, it can be obtained using appropriate methods, but the difficulty and costs of the survey will increase.[18]

5.5. Treatment of results

5.5.1. Average consumption

Food consumption or nutrient intake based on household surveys may be expressed 'per person' or 'per head' over a given period of time, usually a day or a week. The age and sex structure of the family is ignored. Comparisons between households or communities will be valid only if the composition of the groups is similar. This type of analysis may therefore be useful for:

(1) regional comparisons of areas with similar age and sex structure;

(2) comparisons of particular household types in different socio-economic circumstances (e.g. families with two or more children in different income groups);

(3) longitudinal studies of single communities.

5.5.2. Proportion of diet consumed from the household food supply

If individual household members do not record consumption of food obtained away from home, then it may be necessary to know what proportion of the diet is obtained from the household food supply. This is usually done by counting the number of meals eaten at home out of the total possible number in the survey period. As meals will be different sizes, it is necessary to apply a weighting factor in the calculation of the proportion. Table 5.1 gives suggested factors for different meals for a variety of nutrients. These factors are based on a day with 7 meal periods, 4 main meals (breakfast, mid-day meal, evening meal, and late supper) and 3 minor meals (early morning tea, mid-morning break, and mid-afternoon break). The factors show the percentage contribution of each meal to nutrient intake *on the days the meals were eaten.* Each row,

Table 5.1. Average percentage contribution of meals to the daily intake of energy and 11 nutrients on the days the meals were eaten*

Nutrient	Meal						
	Early morning tea	Breakfast	Mid-morning break	Mid-day meal	Mid-afternoon	Evening meal†	Late supper†
Energy	6	20	9	30	10	34	15
Protein	5	19	7	33	7	36	13
Fat	5	17	8	32	9	37	14
Carbohydrate	7	22	10	28	12	31	15
Calcium	10	24	13	26	10	29	18
Iron	2	21	6	33	7	37	12
Retinol equivalents	5	17	7	34	7	37	12
Thiamin	5	33	7	29	6	30	13
Riboflavin	10	32	10	24	8	28	16
Nicotinic acid equivalents	5	24	7	32	6	33	13
Ascorbic acid	6	14	7	36	7	37	13
Dietary fibre	1	25	6	32	7	35	11
Main meals only							
Cambridge	—	20	—	30	—	34	15
National Food Survey	—	21	—	29	—	34	16

*Meals were eaten by 487 subjects aged 0–57 years in Cambridge, England. Rows may add up to more than 100 because not every subject ate all meals, every day.
For main meals only: Cambridge and National Food Survey values.
†Interchangeable according to whichever was the larger meal.

therefore, adds up to more than 100, as not every subject in the study ate every meal every day. Having established a subject's meal pattern, these factors can be used to estimate the *relative* contribution of the different meals to the daily intake. The simplest approach is to base the pattern on the factors for energy. It is important to note, however, that the values for some nutrients are very different from those for energy, and this may need to be considered when interpreting results.

Clearly, these factors are guides only as they are based on a single study of families in Cambridge, England. The bottom two rows show values based on main meals only, the first line from the Cambridge study being based on energy only. The second, from values given in the National Food Survey, is based on energy and protein.[15] In the National Food Survey, the contribution of meals away from home is based on a 4 meal per day pattern, but this may lead to an underestimate of the amount of food consumed away from home. Further analysis of this problem is given in Nelson.[19] This approach can also be used to estimate the proportion of the household food supply consumed by visitors.

5.5.3. Dietary adequacy

The nutrient intake of a family may be compared with the sum of the recommended allowances/intakes (RDA) appropriate to the age and sex of the family members. Allowance must be made for food obtained and eaten away from home, and for food given to visitors or pets, or wasted. Allowances for food eaten away from home can be made by multiplying each subject's RDA by the proportion of their diet consumed from the household food supply (5.5.2). The nutrient content of the household food supply must be adjusted by subtracting:

(1) the proportion consumed by visitors, calculated as for household members on the basis of the number of meals eaten;

(2) the amount given to pets—this should be subtracted before foods are coded for nutrient calculations;

(3) preparation losses;

(4) waste (average from about 4 to 6 per cent).[25]

The adjusted values for the household food supply can then be divided by the sum of the adjusted RDA values to give an estimate of dietary adequacy at the family level. Given the inaccuracies inherent in these calculations, estimates of dietary adequacy should be based on values for at least 20 families.[15]

The main advantage of assessment of dietary adequacy in this way is that it allows households of differing composition to be compared or pooled, assuming that biases in the survey method apply equally to all household types.[1] The underlying assumption in this method of analysis is that nutrients are distributed within the household according to the RDA. If this is not true, then the estimate of adequacy for the household may not apply equally to all household members.

5.5.4. Distribution of foods and nutrients within households

There are many studies which show that foods are not distributed equally within families. Thus, men often receive more than their 'fair share', particularly of energy and protein-rich foods, and young girls generally receive least in relation to their needs. In Latin America it has been shown that in most families some foods are dedicated to the children and others to adults.[9-11] Flores *et al.*[8] suggest that the only way to clarify the food distribution within the household is to carry out a combined study of the total family food consumption and that of individual family members.

Studies in both developed and developing countries have shown that the distribution of nutrients within families is not in line with the RDAs.[3, 5, 21] Thus, the adequacy of diet of particular age/sex groups within families may not be equal to the average for the family as a whole. In theory, this problem can be overcome by using factors to predict how nutrients are distributed within a household. Intakes, according to age and sex, are expressed in relation to that of the male head of household, whose intake is taken as unity. Table 5.2 gives examples of measured family values which show how intakes for energy and 13 nutrients were distributed according to ages and sex.

Having used the factors to predict how nutrients are distributed, the dietary adequacy of different age/sex subgroups can then be calculated separately. In practice, there are two major disadvantages to this approach:

1. The factors used are entirely dependent on the man's level of energy intake. Factors for the families of a group of heavy manual labourers, such as miners, would be much lower than those for a group of sedentary workers, such as office clerks.

2. The factors used for one community will not necessarily apply to another one, apparently similar. Thus, a pilot survey would be required to estimate the factors appropriate to each community. Factors can be determined using the semi-weighed method.[18] This, however, is very labour-intensive for both respondents and fieldworkers and may over-stretch the resources allocated to a straightforward household survey.

Table 5.2. Measured family-values* (distribution factors) for energy and 13 nutrients in 8 age/sex groups in 79 Cambridge families

| Age group (years): | 18 and over | | 11–17 | | 5–10 | | Under 5 | |
Sex:	male	female	male	female	male	female	male	female
Nutrient								
Energy	1.00	0.70	0.91	0.81	0.73	0.61	0.50	0.48
Protein	1.00	0.73	0.84	0.77	0.69	0.56	0.52	0.43
Fat	1.00	0.74	0.89	0.80	0.76	0.60	0.55	0.45
Carbohydrate	1.00	0.71	0.99	0.94	0.84	0.70	0.52	0.52
Calcium	1.00	0.81	0.86	0.82	0.83	0.71	0.81	0.64
Iron	1.00	0.75	0.87	0.77	0.78	0.58	0.52	0.52
Retinol	1.00	1.23	0.67	0.70	1.09	0.59	0.68	0.43
Carotene	1.00	0.95	1.04	1.13	0.95	0.93	0.44	0.48
Thiamin	1.00	0.77	1.07	0.93	1.03	0.74	0.67	0.57
Riboflavin	1.00	0.80	0.95	0.81	0.93	0.71	0.78	0.60
Nicotinic acid	1.00	0.71	0.92	0.76	0.77	0.58	0.46	0.41
Tryptophan/60	1.00	0.73	0.85	0.76	0.70	0.56	0.52	0.41
Ascorbic acid	1.00	1.09	0.80	0.88	0.80	0.62	0.74	0.72
Dietary fibre	1.00	0.80	1.03	0.95	1.02	0.72	0.56	0.58

*Family-value = $\dfrac{\text{Nutrient intake of family member}}{\text{Nutrient intake of male head of household}}$

By definition, therefore, family-value of male head of household equals unity. (Values taken from Nelson[21] q.v. for complete table with SE.)

5.6. Validity and precision

As with other dietary survey methods, there are no absolute standards against which to test the validity and reliability of results from household surveys. All comparisons are therefore in relation to other methods which are also fallible (10.1, 10.2.4).

5.6.1. Food account and inventory methods

The validity of the food accounts method used in the National Food Survey of Great Britain has been examined by Nelson *et al.*[20]
Relative validity was tested by comparing the estimate of energy intake per person per day based on the National Food Survey with the estimated energy requirement. In 1978, the average energy content of the household diet based on the National Food Survey was given as 9.46 MJ (2250 kcal)/person/day. This did not include the 11 per cent of the diet which was obtained from outside the home, providing, in theory, a further 1.17 MJ (280 kcal)/person/day. Energy from sweets, soft drinks, and alcoholic beverages provided an additional 1.40 MJ (335 kcal), yielding a total of 12.02 MJ (2860 kcal)/person/day. Consumption of food by visitors (4 per cent) and waste (6 per cent) would account for 1.20 MJ (285 kcal), leaving an estimated intake of 10.82 MJ (2575 kcal)/person/day. This value of 1.37 MJ (325 kcal) is 14 per cent in excess of the estimated energy requirement of the population, 9.54 MJ (2270 kcal)/person/day.

Relative validity was also tested by comparing the nutrient content of home food purchases, adjusted for consumption by visitors and waste, with that of 7-day semi-weighed records of home food consumption which excluded sweets, soft drinks, and alcoholic beverages. Purchases were between 9 per cent and 16 per cent in excess of measured home consumption for most nutrients. These findings suggest that there is a net increase in purchasing of about 10–15 per cent during food account surveys covering one week. The excess food is probably stored, rather than wasted, or is given to visitors. Other workers, too, have also reported that there may be an initial stocking up during the first week of record keeping.[23]

An important difference in the degree of overpurchasing was observed between income groups. Upper income group families purchased foods which provided on average 11 per cent more energy than measured home food consumption. Lower income group families purchased 20 per cent in excess of consumption. Thus, while the measured home intakes were significantly different between income groups, 7.25 MJ (1725 kcal) compared with 6.49 MJ (1545 kcal)/person/day in the upper and lower income groups, respectively, no such difference was observed when based on purchasing data, 8.08 MJ (1925 kcal) compared with 7.79 MJ (1855 kcal)/person/day. Purchasing data, therefore, may obscure real differences in dietary intake between groups in which the survey bias is different. It is also possible that in this study the lower income group underrecorded their food consumption, although there is no strong evidence to suggest that this occurred.

Estimates of the standard error (SE, 9.2.1) of consumption and expenditure are given for the National Food Survey in Appendix A of the *Annual report of the national food survey committee*.[15] Over all the households ($n=7094$), percentage SE for food consumption ranged from 0.7 per cent for liquid milk and 1.9 per cent for total carcass meat, to 6.3 per cent for oatmeal and oat products and 8.6 per cent for 'branded food drinks'. Estimates of the percentage standard errors of average per capita food consumption for 11 major food categories in all households are given in Table 5.3. Standard errors are also given in the National Food Survey reports by household composition. These values are larger than for all households because of the smaller numbers within each category. For example, for milk, percentage SE ranges from 1.3 per cent for households with 2 adults and no children ($n=2104$) to 6.6 per cent for households with 2 adults and 4 or more children ($n=82$). These errors relate to mean consumption for groups of households based on

Table 5.3. Estimates of the percentage standard errors* of average per caput food consumption, all households, 1984

Food group	Percentage standard error	
	All foods in group	Separate items in group (range)
Milk and cream	0.6	0.7–4.7
Cheese	1.3	1.4–3.9
Meat	1.0	1.1–3.4
Fish	1.6	2.3–5.0
Eggs	1.1	—
Fats	1.2	1.8–3.5
Sugar and preserves	1.5	1.6–2.6
Vegetables	1.0	1.2–1.9
Fruit	1.3	1.4–2.1
Cereals	0.7	1.1–6.3
Beverages	1.5	1.7–8.6

(Values are taken from Ministry of Agriculture, Fisheries and Food, Appendix A, Table 8.15.)
*Formula for percentage errors $= CV/\sqrt{n}$ (CV=coefficient of variation (9.2.1)).

records taken over a 7-day period. It can be seen that with records from a large number of households very precise estimates of apparent consumption can be obtained. There is no data on the week-to-week variation *within* households.

5.6.2. List–recall method

Burk and Pao[2] have reviewed the literature on the validity and reliability of list–recall methods. Evidence quoted from a study of 900 households suggests that the list–recall results are about 20 per cent lower than those obtained by inventory methods.[12] Percentage SE was also less with the list–recall method. Similar findings were shown by the Consumer Panel of the US Office of Price Administration in 1943. In contrast, comparison of list-recall results from the 1965–66 *United States household food consumption survey* with food disappearance data for the same period shows the survey results to be 5–10 per cent greater. The differences vary according to household composition. Thus, studies of relative validity are not consistent.

The validity of the list–recall method has also been tested by assessing the number of items recalled and by using the items stored in the larder to assist recall. Neither of these approaches has done more than illustrate that the quality of the recalled information is as complete as the respondent can make it. It is not evidence that the recalled list is a complete or accurate representation of foods actually used.

Percentage SE from list–recall methods are not dissimilar to values for other household methods when the number of households is large (e.g. 500 or more). As with food account and inventory methods, there is virtually no data on the within-household variation in purchases or intake.

5.6.3. Distribution within households

There is little information on the accuracy of the results concerning the distribution of food and nutrients within households. Nelson[21] has calculated SE for distribution factors within his sample from Cambridge, England, and has stated that 'it is theoretically possible to use family values (distribution factors) to predict the distribution of intake within families'.

He concludes, however: 'Factors which would influence distribution such as activity levels, food wastage, consumption of food by visitors and the proportion of food obtained from outside the household food supply would all need to be taken into account. The cost and difficulty of this exercise would be substantial'. Moreover, using factors to predict distribution may, in itself, obscure problems of over- or under-nutrition within certain age/sex groups within households. They should therefore be used with great caution and any findings based on their use should be supported by more detailed studies of the at-risk group using techniques for the study of individuals (Chapter 6).

References

1. Baines, A. J. H. and Hollingsworth, D. F. (1955). The diets of elderly women living alone. *Proc. Nutr. Soc.* **14**, 77–80.
2. Burk, M. C. and Pao, E. M. (1976). *Methodology for large-scale surveys of household and individual diets.* Home Economics Research Report No. 40, United States Department of Agriculture, Washington DC.
3. den Hartog, A. P. (1972). Unequal distribution of food within the household. *Nutr. Newsletter* **10**, 8–17.
4. Edholm, O. G., Adam, J. M., Healy, M. J. R., Wolff, H. S., Goldsmith, R., and Best, T. W. (1970). Food intake and energy expenditure of army recruits. *Br. J. Nutr.* **24**, 1091–107.
5. Ferro-Luzzi, A., Norgan, N. G., and Paci, C. (1981). An evaluation of the distribution of protein and energy intakes in some New Guinean households. *Nutr. Rep. Intl.* **24**, 153–63.
6. Flores, M. (1962). Dietary studies for the assessment of the nutritional status of population in non-modernized societies. *Am. J. Clin. Nutr.* **11**, 344–55.
7. Flores, M., Garcia, B., Flores, Z., and Lara, M. Y. (1964). Annual patterns of family and children's diet in three Guatemalan Indian villages. *Br. J. Nutr.* **18**, 281–93.
8. Flores, M., Flores, Z., and Lara, M. Y. (1965). Estimation of family and mothers' dietary intake comparing two methods. (San Antonio La Paz, Guatemala). *Trop. Geog. Med.* **17**, 135–45.
9. Flores, M., Menchu, M. T., Lara, M. Y., and Guzman, M. A. (1970). Relacion entre la ingesta de calorias y nutrientes en preescolares y las disponibilidad de alimentos en la familia. *Arch. Latinoam. Nutr.* **20**, 44–58.
10. Flores, M., Menchu, M. T., and Guzman, M. A. (1973). Evaluacion dietetica de familias y pre-escolares mediante la aplicacion de diferentes metodos y tecnicas. *Arch. Latinoam. Nutr.* **23**, 325–44.
11. Flores, M. and Flores, R. (1984). Effects of dependence on seasonally available food. In: *Malnutrition: determinants and consequences.* (While, P. L. and Selvey, N., eds). pp. 207–19. Alan R. Liss, New York.
12. Grossman, E. and Popka, D. Methodology of a household food consumption survey in Cincinnati, Ohio, Nov. 1969–Jan. 1970. (unpublished reference in Burk and Pao, 1976).
13. Hollingsworth, D. F. and Baines, A. H. J. (1961). A survey of food consumption in Great Britain. In: *Family living studies: a symposium.* Studies and reports No. 63. Geneva International Labour Office.
14. Institute of Nutrition of Central America and Panama and Nutrition Program. Center of Disease Control. (1971). *Nutritional evaluation of the population of Central America and Panama.* Regional summary DHEW

Publication No. (HSM) 72–8120. US Departments of Health, Education and Welfare, Washington DC.

15. Ministry of Agriculture, Fisheries, and Food (1986). *Household food consumption and expenditure.* HMSO, London.
16. Ministry of Food. (1951). *The urban working-class household diet, 1940–49.* HMSO, London.
17. National Research Council. (1949). Nutrition surveys, their techniques and value. *Bull. Natl. Res. Counc.* No. 117, Washington DC.
18. Nelson, M. and Nettleton, P. A. (1980). Dietary survey methods. 1. A semi-weighed technique for measuring dietary intake within families. *J. Hum. Nutr.* **34**, 325–48.
19. Nelson, M. (1983). *A dietary survey method for measuring family food purchases and individual nutrient intakes concurrently.* PhD Thesis, University of London.
20. Nelson, M., Dyson, P. A., and Paul, A. A. (1985). Family food purchases and home food consumption: comparison of nutrient contents. *Br. J. Nutr.* **54**, 373–87.
21. Nelson, M. (1986). The distribution of nutrient intake within families. *Br. J. Nutr.* **55**, 267–77.
22. Platt, B. S., Gray, P. G., Parr, E., Baines, A. H. J., Clayton, S., Hobson, E. A., Hollingsworth, D. F., Berry, W. T. C., and Washington, E. (1964). The food purchases of elderly women living alone. *Br. J. Nutr.* **18**, 413–29.
23. Sudman, S. and Ferber, R. (1971). Experiments in obtaining consumer expenditures by diary methods. *Am. Stat. Assoc. J.* **66**, 725–35.
24. United States Department of Agriculture. (1983). *Food consumption: households in the United States, seasons and year 1977–78. Nationwide food consumption survey 1977–78.* Report No. H-6 Washington DC. US Government Printing Office.
25. Wenlock, R. W., Buss, D. H., Derry, B. J., and Dixon, E. J. (1980). Household food wastage in Britain. *Br. J. Nutr.* **43**, 53–70.
26. Woolaway, M. C., Nelson, M., and Herfst, H. (1985). A study of the nutrient content of hospital meals. *Comm. Med.* **7**, 193–97.

6

Methods for data collection at an individual level

SHEILA A. BINGHAM, MICHAEL NELSON,
ALISON A. PAUL, JOHANNA HARALDSDOTTIR,
ELIN BJØRGE LØKEN, AND WIJA A. VAN STAVEREN

Introduction

Chapter 4 discussed the purpose of studies to estimate the adequacy of dietary intake and to investigate the relationship of diet to nutritional status or the development of disease. Such studies require the collection of food consumption data at the individual level. Data collected at one period of time from large numbers of individuals is called 'cross sectional' data. When data are collected from the same individual(s) over a long period of time, often years, it is called 'longitudinal' data. Usually the information needed is about habitual diet while the individual is 'free living' and continuing with a normal lifestyle. Occasionally, however, it may be necessary to assess how strictly a subject is keeping to a prescribed or modified diet, either to assess progress of treatment or to make a diagnosis.

For the design of any study it is essential to decide first on the type of information needed and there are four different types of information.

1. Mean food consumption of a group of individuals (e.g. to assess the level of calcium intake in children having school milk).

2. Mean and distribution of food consumption in a group (e.g. to determine what proportion of a defined population is at risk because of a low vitamin A intake).

3. The relative magnitude of the food consumption of an individual as belonging to a certain third or fifth of the distribution of intakes. Either quantitative or qualitative data might be collected for this type of information. Type 3 information might also be needed for correlation or regression analyses in studies, for example, on the relationship between iron intake and iron deficiency anaemia.

4. The absolute magnitude of the average food consumption of an

individual. This may have a large error which should be reported. This type of information could be used for clinical purposes.

For the data collection of these four types of information, different methods are available and it may be difficult to decide on which one to select. Before making a choice there are four important points to consider. One is the purpose of the study, the second is the accuracy of the methods, the third is the target group, and the fourth is the availability of resources.

In general, methods can be divided into two basic categories. One category collects data recorded at the time of eating (I). The second category collects data about diet eaten in the immediate, recent or distant past (II and III). In this chapter the following methods will be described.

I   Weighed records
     Estimated records
     Observed weighed records
     Records combined with direct analysis.

II   24-hour recall
     Dietary history
     Food frequency

III Retrospective dietary assessments

IV   Combined methods

The validity of each of the methods when used to obtain the four different types of information is discussed in 6.2, 6.3 and 6.4. However, when studying free-living individuals it is difficult to validate any method with certainty because all the methods rely on information supplied by the subjects themselves. This information may not be correct. In the past routine ways of checking the information have been limited and included cross-questioning, examination of reported portion sizes (Chapter 7), and observations done in canteens of schools and institutions.[39,67] Now some independent checks can be made on validity through, for example, the use of 24-hour urinary nitrogen to check on protein intake.[17,54] More recently, the use of the doubly-labelled water technique to check on energy expenditure and therefore indirectly on energy intake, has been used.[87]

It is essential to clarify the purpose of the study so well that it is obvious which type of information is needed. The most cost-effective method must then be found. Some methods will be excluded because they are too inaccurate to fulfil the purpose, are unsuitable for the target group, or are too expensive for the available resources. The remaining methods must then be considered in detail. Their advantages and disadvantages should be balanced against the priorities of the study. It should be considered, for example, whether it is more important to have a high participation rate or more precise information on the weight of foods eaten.

Any method consists of two components: collection of data and conversion into nutrients. This chapter describes the methods to collect the data and critically evaluates when they can be used.

The information given should help in making a suitable choice of the method to be used.

Chapter 8 discusses the conversion of data into energy and nutrients whereas Chapter 14 gives guidance for practical implementation. Estimates of the costs, in terms of time and resources associated with each method, are discussed in Chapter 13.

6.1. Weighed records (3.2.8)

6.1.1. Principles

In the weighed record technique or method, the subject is taught to weigh and record the food and its weight immediately before eating and to weigh any leftovers.[116] However, not every item of food needs to be weighed. Where weighing would interfere with normal eating habits, it is usual to accept a descriptive record of the foods consumed, for example, in a restaurant, from which the weights of foods are estimated by the nutritionist investigator.[13, 70] Details of recipes are necessary and a data bank of average recipes used in a particular locality greatly simplifies the procedure.[83, 119] (Chapters 8 and 13). This method is very different from the so-called 'precise weighing' which is necessary if food composition tables with values for cooked foods are not available. Raw ingredients, the cooked food, meal, or snack, plus the individual portions must all be weighed,[84] and aliquots for chemical analysis may also be necessary (6.4). It is usual for skilled fieldworkers to carry out this type of survey, rather than the subjects themselves (Chapter 13).

6.1.2. Practical aspects

The weighed record is thought to be the most accurate method of dietary assessment, but it needs to be used with care. If habitual diet is being assessed, it must be stressed that 'usual' diet is being investigated and that the subject must not use the opportunity, for example, to restrict energy intake. Further, in order to avoid bias in response it is an advantage not to disclose the precise nutrient of interest being studied. Randomly selected population groups, in particular, need to be given simple verbal and written instructions and a demonstration of how foods should be weighed, preferably in the home. Table 6.1 is one example of a diary of events for a weighed dietary survey (Chapter 14).

Table 6.1. Diary of recruitment and visits for a weighed record dietary survey

Day	Events
3–6 weeks beforehand	Explain the survey and obtain cooperation from influential members of the population to be studied. Prepare posters, advertisements, and media contacts if necessary. Obtain collaboration from clinical staff if patients are to be studied. Randomly select subjects from the population, medical, or electoral registers. Obtain and prepare scales, notebooks, pens, demonstration foods, transport, computer database of nutrient information, and questionnaires.
1 week beforehand	Recruit selected subjects (e.g. at a clinic, hospital, or school). A letter sent beforehand, together with a newspaper article or endorsement from an influential member of the community, helps recruitment of randomly selected population samples. The letter should suggest a time for a visit at home to ask for his/her help. When cooperation is obtained, make a date for the survey to start.
The day before	Visit the subject, or ask him/her to visit the clinic, when convenient for him/her. Demonstrate the principles in a simple way using demonstration foods. Ask the subjects to repeat the demonstration, writing down the weights in the record book, and to practise with the evening meal.
The first day	Check the practice record and the meals weighed out so far. Make sure that the weights look reasonable and, if not, ask the subject to weigh out a similar portion for you to check. If the subject has understood the method, ask for details to be added to the record, referring to the instructions (Table 6.2). Emphasize that the subject must not change his/her usual dietary habits; if necessary (e.g. when occasionally eating out) a record of place, cost, description, and approximate portion size will suffice.
Other survey days	Revisit the subject if necessary.
Day after survey	Check the complete record for errors, omissions, and doubtful data. Explain that you may have to visit the subject again or to telephone if there are any further queries. Thank the subject for his/her cooperation and, if possible or appropriate, give a small gift.

Table 6.1. (*cont.*)

Day	Events
	Code or calculate the records as soon as possible after visiting the subject.
After the survey is completed	Follow up with press reports on the general results, and give the subjects appropriate individual results if they have asked for them. It is advisable not to offer to make individual results available to a subject at the start or midway through a survey, as this may bias food habits whilst the record is being kept.

Scales

Scales should be robust, accurate to at least ± 5 g and weigh up to 1.5 kg so that a normal plate can be used when weighing the food to be eaten. The 'cumulative weight' technique should be used.[69, 70] In this, the subject records the weight of the plate, then plate weight plus the first food item, followed by the plate weight plus the first and second food item, and so on. Alternatively, with care, a tare might be used (7.1.1). The weights of foods need not be recorded by hand. They can be done verbally. Figure 7.1 shows an electronic scale being used by a subject under study, for such a purpose.

Record book and instructions

When the subject has given a practical demonstration and shown that the principles of the technique have been understood and can be used, the fieldworker can go on to explain the record book in detail. Record books (Fig. 14.2) should be simple, clear, and of a manageable size to be portable and not take up too much room on any kitchen surface. A sample of guidelines for weighing is shown in Table 6.2.

When the subject uses the technique with more confidence it can be explained how more details of the foods eaten can be recorded. These include the kind of meat eaten, how the potatoes were cooked, the type of bread used and recipe details. This can be done conveniently on the first day of weighing, if the subject has by then understood the technique. Most subjects can then be left with instructions to continue for the rest of the survey period, provided that they know where to contact the fieldworker or the clinic if they have any problems. Some subjects, however, may need repeated visits and assistance throughout (7.2.2).

Checking

On the final visit immediately after the subject has completed the survey, the record should be checked in detail and the subject thanked. The records should be coded for computer calculation or calculated by hand

Table 6.2. Guidelines for weighing

Thank you for helping us. It is important that we know exactly what you have eaten. Please weigh and record *everything* you eat and drink (including water). Write down what you have to eat or drink, giving as much detail as you can about each item. For instance, whether bread is white, brown, or wholemeal; whether fruit is eaten peeled or unpeeled; whether meat is fatty or lean, roasted, stewed, or grilled. Give the number of cups of tea or coffee, slices of bread, rashers of bacon, eggs, biscuits, and sweets.

Recipes for any special dish are very helpful, and can be written on the form.

Remember to write down

- anything you eat away from home; cups of tea (say whether you had milk and/or sugar);
- between-meal snacks or nibbles while cooking;
- beer, sherry, or other alcoholic drinks;
- sweets and chocolates;
- fruit;
- crisps and nuts.

To weigh your food

- if you are going to eat a hot meal, warm a suitable plate while you are cooking your food;
- record the time of day in the 'Time' column on the form provided, and place your plate or cup on the scale, recording the weight in the 'Wt served' column;
- place one item of food on the plate or in the cup, record the weight in the 'Wt served' column, and fill in the 'Food' column;
- add the next item of food and record the total weight. Repeat until you have served out your meal.

Please record each item of food on a separate line.

Should the scale zero need correcting, turn the screw at the back of the scale a little to adjust it.

If you have not eaten all the food on your plate, or if there is waste, like bones:

- put another plate on the scale and record its weight;
- place one item of waste or left food on the plate and record the weight in the 'left-overs' column, and fill in the 'Food' column;
- add the next item and record the total weight. Repeat until you have weighed out all the food and waste left.

Start a new page for each day and use as many pages as you need.

Enter the date and day of the week on every page.

Please do not fill in any of the other spaces or calculate the actual weight of each food item.

If you have any queries, please ring ....

as soon as possible, but certainly within a few days, in order that the subject can be contacted again, if necessary, to answer queries. Coding should be checked by a different fieldworker before entering the record into a computer.

6.1.3. Uses, examples, and limitations

The weighed record is suitable for use in any literate population, including hospital patients, volunteers, and randomly selected population samples. In theory, and given certain provisos, it is appropriate for all four types of dietary information (6.1.4). Because of its probable greater accuracy, it is usually the required method in research. It is also a preferred method for multicentre studies wanting types 1 and 2 information because technical instructions can be standardized easily and possible biases are avoided from estimations of weights of food and frequency of food consumption. This method has been used in Britain to study large groups of children, the elderly and adults,[6,37,42,106] and it has also been used in international collaborative studies.[53,60,66]

The weighed record cannot be used for some disabled or illiterate subjects. It requires a higher degree of cooperation from subjects than some other methods because, when keeping weighed records, the subjects do most of the dietary survey work themselves. This is likely to affect the response from the randomly selected samples unless great care is taken. Eighty per cent response rates are essential for types 1 and 2 information[50] and have been obtained with the weighed record.[13,42,50,53,106]

Weighed dietary surveys do have a greater risk of bias, though it is not as great as is sometimes suggested.[77] Persistence in recruiting, payment, or gifts in return for the subject's time, as is done in other research studies, and the involvement of local organizations, the press, radio, or television are all vital for the success of epidemiological studies.

6.1.4. Accuracy

While it is generally assumed that the weighed food record is the most accurate dietary assessment method to use for free living individuals,[71] no objective evidence for this assumption is given in the early literature. Validity and precision, the two factors in accuracy, will be considered separately.

In general, it is easier to validate group results (types 1 and 2 information) than individual data (types 3 and 4). However, when information of types 3 and 4 is required, it is particularly important to consider precision.

To improve accuracy, study design must randomize the study days.

This takes into account the seasonal, as well as weekday *versus* weekend, variations in dietary intakes between groups (types 1 and 2) and between individuals (types 3 and 4).

6.1.5. Validity

It is difficult to validate dietary survey methods in free-living individuals. A potential validation method is to compare the daily protein intake with the 24-hour urinary nitrogen.[17, 54]

With individual subjects having a stable body weight, confidence in the dietary data is possible if the urinary nitrogen from an 8-day collection of 24-hour samples of urine is 81 ± 5 per cent of the dietary nitrogen intake.[17] However, the samples must be complete.[15]

A study on a small group of volunteers compared the doubly-labelled water technique, which is an independent measure of energy expenditure with records of food intake. Results suggested that, in this population of normal weights, data from weighed records of dietary intake agreed with energy expenditure.[88, 89]

However, in obese women, energy intake, as recorded, was about 2 MJ (465 kcal) lower than actual energy expenditure. This study was small, but it supports other studies' conclusions that obese people do not report their habitual food intake.[104,113] Recent studies suggest that in individuals, living in industrialized countries, average 24-hour energy expenditure exceeds 24-hour basal metabolic rate by a factor of 1.3.[87] Revised calculations allow greater confidence to be placed on predicted basal metabolic rate if body weight is known.[95] Using these rates, for larger groups of normal weight volunteers and randomly selected populations, results show that average energy intakes, as assessed from the weighed record technique, are 1.3 to 1.4 times the predicted basal metabolic rate in women and 1.3 to 1.8 in men.[12,13,53,106,115,121]

In the case of individuals, tables cannot be used to predict basal metabolic rate (and hence energy expenditure) because there is a 12 per cent individual variation in basal metabolic rate and the energy expenditure of very active individuals may be at least twice the 24-hour basal metabolic rate.[120] Nevertheless, reported habitual energy intakes less than three standard deviations away from the predicted basal metabolic rate times 1.2 (for example, 5 MJ (1090 kcal) for women and 7.5 MJ (1785 kcal) for men), are without doubt erroneously low.

6.1.6. Precision

Precision or reproducibility of a method is the extent to which it produces the same results, when repeated in the same situation (3.4.3). In the majority of types 1 and 2 studies, where the average dietary intake of a group of subjects is assessed, subjects are asked to continue recording for 7 days. If only types 1 and 2 data are required, this has no statistical justification. Statistically it is preferable and more cost-effective to make single observations on a large number of individuals rather than a large number of observations on a few individuals. However, when subjects have been taught how to keep a record, there is good reason for obtaining more than a single day's record from each individual. If this is done it would then be possible to study variable nutrients such as dietary fibre, cholesterol, calcium, or polyunsaturated fatty acids. For these highly variable nutrients, which have coefficients of variation of 60 per cent or more, the within-person variation becomes important in deter-mining the power to which a given sample size can detect a difference in the mean. Table 6.3 illustrates this point.

Table 6.3. Detectable difference*† in means for sample size of 500, $\alpha = 0.05$, $\beta = 0.20$

	Percentage detectable difference in averages from different numbers of observations on each subject		
	1 day	3 days	7 days
Energy	6	5	4
Protein	6	5	5
Fat	7	5	5
Dietary fibre	7	5	5
Riboflavin	8	5	4

*Variances: Bingham et al.[13]
†Formulas: Ducimetiere,[38] Cole and Black[35]

: $S = \sqrt{\sigma_B^2 (1 + \sigma_W^2/k\sigma_B^2)}$

where σ_B^2 = between-person variance
σ_W^2 = within-person variance
k = number of records

: Difference = $\sqrt{2 (2.8 \times S)^2/n}$

where n = sample size, $\alpha = 0.05$, $\beta = 0.20$.

It can be seen that with a sample size of 500 only a 6–8 per cent differ-ence in the means would be detectable if a single day's record were obtained, but with a 3-day record a difference of 5 per cent could be detected for all the nutrients to be investigated. However, there is little statistical justification in extending the numbers of records beyond 3 days, for example, to 7 days. A record for a single day may also incur greater risk since any change in food habits would introduce bias into the results. In general therefore, a 3-day record, randomized to cover seasonal and weekday variations is recommended for types 1 and 2 data.

With individual dietary assessments (types 3 and 4) because of day-to-day variation in food and nutrient intake, the precision is low unless the numbers of observations on each individual are increased. Thus, 3–4 days of observation are recommended for group averages. However, depending on the nutrient of interest and the desired level of precision, more observations are necessary for the individual.

Table 6.4 shows the numbers of days of observation required for type 4 data with a precision of ±10 per cent standard error of the mean for various nutrients based on the average daily variations shown in Table 6.5. It can be seen (in Table 6.4) that at this level of precision, a 7-day record is sufficient to measure only energy, carbohydrate, and protein.

A larger margin of error is introduced into the measurement of other nutrients (Table 6.4) when individuals are observed for only 7 days, lessening the correlation coefficient between dietary and other biological variables (Chapter 10).[96] For these more variable nutrients therefore, a minimum of 14 days of observation is required if a standard error of ±10 per cent is the desired average level of precision (Table 6.4). Observations do not need to be made over consecutive days. They can be split up into 3- or 4-day periods over the year and randomized to allow for weekends and seasonal variations.

Some subjects have stable food habits and therefore within-person (daily) coefficients of variation are less than the average shown in Table

Table 6.4. Number of days of observation required for individual data

Item	Average per cent standard error* (% SE) of a 7-day record	Number of days* of records necessary to be within 10 per cent of the mean intake
Energy	9	5
Carbohydrate	9	6
Protein	10	7
Fat	12	10
Dietary fibre	12	10
Calcium	12	10
Iron	13	12
Thiamin	15	15
Riboflavin	17	19
Cholesterol	20	27
Vitamin C	23	36

*Calculated from Balogh et al.[5]:

$\% SE = CV/\sqrt{k} = 0.378 \times CV$

$k = CV^2/(\% SE)^2 = 0.01 \times CV^2$

and CV from Table 6.5.

$\% SE = (SE/mean) \times 100\%$
$CV = (SD/mean) \times 100\%$
$k =$ number of records.

6.5. They can be observed for shorter periods. Longer investigations would always be necessary for those with erratic eating habits. Table 6.6 shows the theoretical number of daily records required to measure dietary intakes to the same level of precision in 90 per cent of individuals within a population.

Table 6.7 shows the number of recording days necessary to classify subjects into thirds of the distribution for type 3 information in epidemiological studies. This is based on data from three population groups. In any specific population the actual numbers of records will depend on the specific ratio of daily variation to between-person variation. Nevertheless, it is clear from Table 6.7 that whereas a 7-day

Table 6.5. Within person variation (percentage) of energy and selected nutrients, from 19 population samples

Item	Average* within-person variation (%)	Range* in within-person variation (%)
Energy	23	4–45
Carbohydrate	25	7–52
Protein	27	9–52
Fat	31	11–69
Dietary fibre	31	14–61
Calcium	32	17–78
Iron	35	18–84
Thiamin	39	10–85
Riboflavin	44	12–101
Cholesterol	52	8–121
Vitamin C	60	15–177

*Data from up to 19 population samples in Britain, USA, Canada, and Israel (Bingham[18]).

Table 6.6. Number of days required to determine the mean intake of individual subjects* with a standard error of ± 10 per cent or less

Nutrient	Number of days† for:		
	50% of population	70% of population	90% of population
Energy	5	7	13
Protein	5	7	14
Fat	9	13	23
Non starch polysaccharides	12	18	28

*Randomly selected Cambridgeshire men 20–80 years ($n=32$) (Bingham *et al.*[12]).
†Formula $k = CV^2/(\% \text{ SE})^2$ (Balogh *et al.*[5]).

Table 6.7. Number of recording days required to classify correctly 80 per cent of men into thirds of the distribution†

	British Civil Servants (Marr[72])	Random selection of British men (Bingham et al.[12])	Random selection of Swedish men* (Callmer[31])
Energy	7	5	7
Protein	6	5	7
Fat	9	9	7
Carbohydrate	4	3	3
Sugar	2	2	—
Dietary fibre	6	10	—
P:S ratio	11	—	—
Cholesterol	18	—	—
Alcohol	4	—	14
Vitamin C	—	6	14
Thiamin	—	6	15
Riboflavin	—	10	—
Calcium	—	4	5
Iron	—	12	9

*Callmer (personal communication). 58×7-day records from middle-aged men randomly selected in Stockholm, Sweden.

†For an individual in the lower third of the distribution, the probability of being classified in the upper third is 20 per cent or less, and *vice versa* (Liu et al.[65]).

record is probably sufficient to classify thirds of the distribution for energy and energy-yielding nutrients, longer periods are necessary for items such as alcohol, some vitamins and minerals, and cholesterol. However, if less precision is acceptable and classification into extreme fifths of the distribution is needed, a 7-day record would be sufficient even for these more variable food constituents.[65, 78]

6.2. Estimated records (3.2.9)

6.2.1. Principles

For this method subjects are taught to keep records, in portion sizes, of all the foods they eat on each day of the study. The portion sizes are described in household measures using the utensils commonly found in their homes. These might include spoons or ladles, tea or coffee cups, glasses or bottles (7.1.2). The investigator quantifies these household measures by volume. The approximate weights of the foods used can then be determined by weighing duplicate portions. Weights can also be determined by using knowledge of the food densities. This is the volume of the food divided by its weight (dl/g). Weighing scales are not used by subjects in this method.

6.2.2. Practical aspects

The design of the form, a number of which are usually kept in a record book, depends on:

- the aim of the study;
- the kind of information required;
- the expected accuracy of the measurements made.

They should be pre-tested in a small pilot study. As described in 6.1.2 record books should be of a convenient size. Depending on the nature of the study and the preference of the investigators, the record form may be of the closed or open type (Chapter 14).

A closed form is a pre-coded record form listing all of the commonly eaten foods in units of specified portion sizes, arranged in groups each of which has a similar nutrient composition.[58] Subjects are asked to indicate how many items of each food are eaten each day and space is provided to describe any foods eaten but not listed on the form. This technique allows rapid coding, using food composition tables, and computer calculation for energy and nutrient intake. However, this form could be restricted as it requires subjects to describe the foods eaten in defined units which may be unfamiliar.

An open form is used more often because there are no restrictions as no descriptions of portion sizes are given. Subjects are asked to describe on this form all the foods eaten each day by using either the measures provided by the investigators[75] or their own household utensils.[77] This form would take longer to code the foods eaten, but accuracy would be gained when calculating energy and nutrient intakes.

Distribution and collection of records

Estimated records are particularly well suited for collecting cross-sectional data. For sample size and number of days per person needed see 6.1.6 and Chapter 10. Distribution and collection of records might be done as described for the weighed records. However, since scales are not used there are two other possibilities:

(1) Record books with clear instructions can be posted to the subjects. To encourage cooperation in the study and confirm its purpose, it is an advantage to send with the instructions a letter from a known and respected person such as the family doctor. A single interview is then all that is necessary to collect and check the record. This approach is especially useful if a 24-hour record is required from a large number of subjects, for example for type 1 information.

(2) Instead of posting the record books and instructions, they could be given to the subjects who are trained individually or in groups, before the study begins. This, however, can be costly in terms of interviewer time especially if 24-hour records from many subjects are required for the study. As before, a final interview would be necessary for the collection and checking of the records (Table 13.1).

Portion sizes and determination of weights

Portion sizes are best described in terms of the subject's own household utensils. Any measuring utensils provided by the investigator could alter usual serving habits. Descriptions in terms of standard portions should not be used unless they are familiar and widely used in the study area, because both these factors could affect the accuracy of records.

Descriptions of portions given by the subjects are used to compile a set of food weights and densities. This involves a great deal of 'back up' work for the investigator especially in the initial stages of using estimated records and is discussed in detail in 13.4. If subjects describe foods in standard measures, this work is reduced considerably but some accuracy is lost.

Guidelines for determining the weights of portions are given in Table 6.8. They relate to studies in which the subject's own household utensils are used to describe portion sizes. The guidelines also apply to situations where the foods are served separately to each person in individual portions. To obtain maximum information about diets in which foods are served in this way, the following points should be considered:

1. Allow subjects to describe portions in terms of their own household utensils.
2. Measure the volume of all the utensils used.
3. Ask the subject, if willing, to serve out specimen portions in their own kitchen to allow the investigator to collect the weights of these foods. These might be slices of bread, bowls of rice, or spoons of sugar used in drinks.
4. Allow some use of weights of foods given on labels and packets. Along with a description of the portion eaten, these weights could be useful records.
5. Never let the subject guess weights which are then entered in the record. These could be very inaccurate and without a description it would be impossible for the investigator to confirm or estimate a portion weight.
6. Use food models or replicas (7.1.3) to help in checking the size of portion used.

When foods are eaten from one, or more than one communal pot or bowl, the difficulty of recording an individual intake in household measures is greatly increased. Nevertheless the following points could be considered:

1. Count the number of times a subject takes food from a communal pot.

2. If possible, estimate the average weight of a 'take'. This can be done later, if food is available, by asking the subject to measure out ten 'takes' which the investigator can then weigh.

Meals, however, are not always homogeneous mixtures of foods, as for example in a stew of meat and vegetables. The composition of each 'take' would vary. Estimating the weights of each food in each portion would be very inaccurate. In these circumstances an alternative method of dietary assessment would be necessary.

6.2.3. Uses, examples, and limitations

Many investigators, particularly in the United States, have used estimated records of diets in prospective studies. The main advantages of the household measures method are that:

(1) it is simpler and less demanding for subjects than the weighing method;

(2) allows rapid and low cost assessment of diets from large numbers of subjects, because scales are not needed;

(3) cooperation rates are likely to be higher than for weighed surveys, especially over long recording periods.[77]

The main disadvantage of using household measures is the loss of accuracy when compared with weighed portions. For groups, the error may be small and of little importance, but for individuals, it may be large (6.2.4).

Household measure records are well suited to the collection of either type 1 or 2 information. These records are as useful as weighed records. Although estimated records are less accurate than weighed records of individuals' diets for type 3 information, they have the same order of accuracy when ranking subjects into thirds or fifths. Estimated records are less suitable for type 4 information than weighed records. However, where the aim is to obtain a record of usual intake in a prospective study, estimated records may be preferable. This is because there is less interference with usual dietary practices if the foods do not need to be weighed. In some situations scales would be inappropriate for individual use (e.g. in illiterate communities or if recording periods are prolonged or where, because of restricted resources, scales cannot be provided).

Table 6.8. Guidelines for determining portion weights (adapted from Nelson and Nettleton[77])

Food	Logbook entry		Determination of weight of a portion*
	Description of food	Description of portion	
1. Commercial foods in individual portions: beefburgers, sausages, fish fingers, fish cakes; cold meats, individual meat pies; cans of sardines, pilchards; individual cakes, pies, puddings, yogurts; biscuits (sweet and savoury); chocolate bars, sweets; packets of crisps, nuts; baby foods.	Brand, manufacturer's name of food; weight or size on label, or price.	Number of items eaten.	Corresponding items purchased, cooked where necessary and weighed in experimental kitchen.
2. Commercial foods in multiple portions; tinned meat or fish; tinned soup, beans, vegetables, fruit, puddings; large meat pies; cakes and pies; made-up jellies or convenience foods; baby foods.	Brand, manufacturer's name of food; weight or size on label, or price.	Fraction of whole. Number of spoonfuls or slices.	Total weight × described fraction. Total weight ÷ total number of spoonfuls or slices served.
3. Spaghetti.	Spaghetti, boiled.	Fraction of total amount cooked.	(Equivalent total amount of uncooked spaghetti weighed by investigator in household or experimental kitchen) × (cooking gains) × described fraction.

4. Pasta other than spaghetti; boiled rice; porridge.	Name of food.	Number of spoonfuls.	(Equivalent total amount of uncooked food weighed by investigator in household or experimental kitchen) × (cooking gains) ÷ total number of spoonfuls served.
5. Breakfast cereals.	Brand, name of cereal.	Number of spoonfuls or bowlfuls.	Equivalent measure of food weighed by investigator in household or experimental kitchen.
6. Breads: wrapped, sliced.	Brand, type of bread (white, brown, etc.), size of loaf, thickness of slice.	Number of slices.	Corresponding items purchased and weighed.
unsliced.	Size of loaf, shop where purchased, type of bread.	Number and thickness of slices.	Subject cut and investigator weighed representative slices *or* investigator purchased corresponding item, cut and weighed slices experimentally.
homemade.	Size of loaf, type of bread.	Number and thickness of slices.	Subject cut and investigator weighed representative slices.
rolls, buns, pastries.	Name and type of roll; description of bun or pastry; shop where purchased.	Number of items eaten.	Corresponding items purchased and weighed.
toasted items.	Description of item, toasted.	As above.	Item toasted by subject and weighed by investigator *or* purchased and toasted and weighed by investigator *or* weight calculated from weight of untoasted item minus experimental cooking losses.

Table 6.8. (*cont.*)

Food	Logbook entry		Determination of weight of a portion*
	Description of food	Description of portion	
7. Milk, cream, tea, coffee, other beverages; gravy, other liquids; yogurt.	Name of food.	Fraction of a pint. Number of spoonfuls, glasses, cups or mugs.	As described. Utensil volumes measured.
8. Cheese.	Names of cheese.	Number and dimensions of pieces.	Volume calculated from dimensions, weight determined from densities.
9. Eggs.	Method of preparation, size.	Number and size eaten.	Different sizes purchased, shelled, and weighed in experimental kitchen. Theoretical cooking losses subtracted.
10. Meat, offal, fish, fowl.	Name of animal, cut of meat, method of preparation, lean or fat.	Number of dimensions of slices.	Volume, calculated from dimensions, weight determined from densities. Total cooked weight (raw weight from purchased data) minus cooking losses minus inedible wastage[a] ÷ total number of slices served.
		Portion (e.g. leg of chicken).	Weight of bought portion (from purchase data) minus cooking losses minus inedible wastage. Total cooked weight (e.g. raw

	Description	Portion/Quantity	Method
	Name of animal, cut of meat, method of preparation, lean or fat.	Portion (e.g. lamb chop, bacon rasher).	weight of whole chicken from purchase data minus cooking losses minus inedible wastage) × theoretical portion fraction.[a] Weight of bought portion (from purchase data or corresponding item purchased and weighed) minus cooking losses minus inedible wastage.[a]
11.	Vegetables.	Name of vegetable, method of preparation.	Number of spoonfuls or pieces.	Total weighed from purchase data (or corresponding items weighed in kitchen or purchased and weighed) minus cooking losses[a] ÷ number of spoonfuls served or pieces prepared.
12.	Fruit, raw.	Name of fruit.	Number of pieces eaten.	Corresponding items weighed in kitchen or purchased and weighed or total from purchase data weight ÷ number of pieces purchased.
13.	Homemade soups, stews, casseroles; cheese, and egg dishes in sauce.	Recipe name.	Number of ladles or spoonfuls.	Total cooked weight calculated from recipe (raw ingredients minus cooking losses[b]) ÷ total number of ladles or spoonfuls served.

Table 6.8. (*cont.*)

Food	Logbook entry		Determination of weight of a portion*
	Description of food	Description of portion	
14. Homemade quiches, pies, cakes; puddings, souffles, mousses; stewed fruit.	Recipe name.	Fraction of whole.	Total cooked weight calculated from recipe (raw ingredients minus cooking losses[b]) × described fraction.
		Number of spoonfuls or slices.	Total cooked weight ÷ total number of spoonfuls or slices served.
15. Sugar.	Type of sugar.	Number of spoonfuls.	10 spoonfuls measured out by subject and weighed by investigator.
16. Sauces and pickles.	Name of food.	Number of spoonfuls.	Equivalent measure of food weighed by investigator in household or experimental kitchen.
		Each use indicated by a tick (√).	Total amount used (weighing container at beginning and end of survey period) minus amounts used in cooking ÷ number of times used during week.
17. Butter, margarine, jam, marmite, other spreads.	Name of spread.	Each use indicated by a tick, associated with the food on which it was spread.	Total amount used (weigh the container at beginning and end of survey period) minus amounts used in

cooking ÷ number of times used during the week. Factors were used to take into account different sizes of slices.

Weight served = average weight × number of times it was used.

Large bread loaf 1.0
Small loaf, rolls, teacake 0.75
Crackers, scones, French bread, malt loaf 0.5
Butter and margarine only; Toasted items: factors above × 1.5.

Subject put usual amount of spread on tip of knife, investigator weighed.

Corresponding items purchased and weighed.

18. Take-away foods.

Name of food, shop where purchased, price.

Number of portions, stated size.

*All weights in this column are determined from: purchase data OR by investigator weighing items in household kitchen OR purchasing and weighing corresponding items.
a Cooking losses, inedible wastage and theoretical portion fractions taken from Paul & Southgate,[83] US Dept. of Agriculture,[127,128] Paul et al.[126]
b Cooking losses calculated experimentally, based on given recipes.

6.2.4. Validity

In the past investigators have validated the estimated record against the weighed record method for type 1 and type 2 information. For groups: the differences in energy and nutrient intakes estimated by the two methods were between 5 and 12 per cent depending on the type of nutrient and population studied.[22,25,40,47,52,123]

Recently Nettleton *et al.*[79] found smaller differences of 2–5 per cent in a validation study. They concluded that the increased use of pre-packed foods improved the reliability of estimated records for estimating group intakes. Furthermore the accuracy can be improved by weighing the foods used frequently each day, for example, spoons of sugar in drinks and fat used on bread.

For individuals, the proportion of individuals' intakes assessed by estimated records that come within ± 10 per cent of the weighed values are shown in Table 6.9.

Table 6.9. Percentage of subjects whose nutrient intakes estimated from household measures is within ± 10 per cent of the value based on weighed records of consumption

Nutrient	Study		
	Bransby *et al.*[25]	Eppright *et al.*[40]	Nettleton *et al.*[79]
Energy	71	33	92
Protein	49	41	87
Fat	41	37	71
Carbohydrate	82	37	89
Calcium	69	35	100
Iron	35	—	84
Thiamin	—	32	87
Ascorbic acid	—	29	79
Number of subjects	49	25	38

(−) indicates value not published.

These results suggest that there may be considerable error in the estimate of individuals' absolute nutrient intakes based on household measures, assuming that the weighed values are correct. However, the inaccuracies of individuals' intakes based on estimated records may be relatively unimportant if the ranking of subjects, using either method, remains the same.[21, 25, 40, 79, 107, 124] The error introduced by the use of household measures in ranking subjects for type 3 information, will result in 15–20 per cent of the subjects being classified in adjacent thirds and less than 1 per cent in opposite thirds when compared with values obtained from weighed records.[78] Where this level of error is acceptable, estimated records provide a suitable alternative to weighing for the ranking of individuals according to their nutrient intakes.

6.2.5. Precision

The number of records needed depends, among other factors, on the type of information needed and has been described in 6.1.6. Because estimated records are less accurate than weighed records, both the between- and within-person variation will be higher. However, in prospective studies it is probably better to use estimated records for assessment of group means, type 1 information, despite the small increase in the number of subjects needed, compared with a weighed record survey.

For ranking of individuals, type 3 information, a similar number of observations will be needed from each subject whether the records are estimated or weighed. The choice of the method to use then depends on the resources available.

6.3. Observed weighed records (3.2.9)

6.3.1. Principles

In situations where the subjects are not able to keep food records themselves, this method requires the active participation of fieldworkers present at each meal. Such situations would occur for example in hospitals or other institutions and in the rural areas of many developing countries, where the level of literacy is low. Here the fieldworkers need to be acceptable to the community, to converse in the local language, and to be able to make correct recordings and descriptions of food items in the language of the principal investigators. These and other problems have been admirably covered by Rutishauser[94] when assessing the methods of measuring food intake in infants and young children in developing countries.

6.3.2. Practical aspects

The following method is used as an example of the observed weighed method. It has been developed over a number of years in the village of Keneba in The Gambia. It was used to measure the food intake of infants and young children and later extended to include all the pregnant and lactating women in the village.[86]

The intake of each mother was measured on the same day each week throughout pregnancy and for 18 months of lactation, and the infant similarly from 1 to 18 months.

The method was suitable for this particular subsistence farming community as the normal eating pattern was two meals a day plus a limited range of well-defined food items taken between meals.

The method used by the fieldworker, to weigh and record the foods to be eaten, is shown in Fig. 6.1.

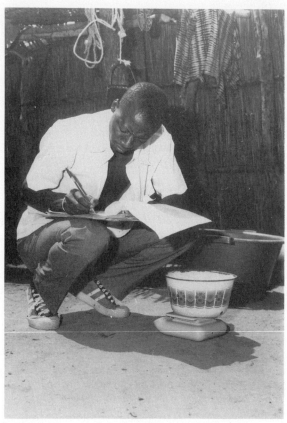

Fig. 6.1. A fieldworker recording a weighed amount of food in the village of Keneba, The Gambia.

The food intake was measured by the fieldworkers who visited the women three times a day to coincide with meal times (although breakfast was rarely taken). Each part of the meal was served into a previously weighed bowl and weighed at each stage. For infants it was normal to make a small bowl of cereal gruel once a day and keep it to give at intervals throughout the day. With the adults, however, a change had to be made in the usual eating habits of a shared food bowl. The woman under study was asked to serve her portion separately. Small portable scales weighing up to 2 kg were used. The fieldworker returned 30 mins to 1 hour later at the end of the meal to weigh the empty bowl or any left-overs that might be eaten later or given to another family member. The name of the food item was entered in the local language on the record form and the food code was added later. At each visit the fieldworker also asked the mother what other foods she or the child had eaten since the last visit. This was estimated by recall (e.g. so many handfuls of groundnuts, a given number of mangoes or oranges, or handfuls or spoonfuls of food from another family's meal). The investigators had previously weighed numerous handfuls of groundnuts and meals and also many mangoes and oranges, and the mean weights multiplied by the frequency of eating were added to the record. When the women were working in the field during the farming season, the fieldworkers visited them there. If it was not possible to do this, the meal that would be taken to the fields was weighed before the women left home.

As there were no available data on the composition of the foods, samples of food were taken at the time of the visits and analysed in the UK for the construction of a local nutrient database (Chapter 8).

This example used for an observed weighed record is in fact a combination of a weighed record and the recall method. Such combinations are not unusual.

Other studies have used an observed precise weighing record in which all the food was weighed before and after cooking, as well as the subject's portion of it. In addition the between meal snacks were weighed.[68,109]

Where meals or snacks are obtained from outside the home, for example from street vendors, the task of the fieldworker is made easier. Either the individual portions brought home can be weighed[73] or equivalent portions can be purchased, weighed, and used in conjunction with a 24-hour recall.[1] Recipes of the vendor's snacks are often well known, but if they are not analyses of them are necessary.

The observed weighed record is commonly used in Norway and Denmark in hospitals and institutions to estimate food intake from bedridden patients, elderly or mentally handicapped subjects, and children in day care centres. The method is often combined with a recall to cover between-meal foods not provided by the caretaker. Foods are weighed after the trays are returned. Fieldworkers are trained nutritionists, dietitians, and sometimes nurses.[51]

In summary the practical aspects to be considered for an observed weighed record are:

(1) availability of skilled fieldworkers acceptable to the target group;

(2) time schedule for the fieldworkers adapted to the eating habits of the subjects;

(3) adequate scales (7.1.1);

(4) easy record books (14.2.1);

(5) availability of a local food composition table or nutrient database.

The examples used for an observed weighed record in fact are a combination of an observed weighed record and a recall method.

6.3.3. Advantages and limitations

The information obtained in the examples given are most suitable for type 1 needs, but it could be used for the other three types, although with less precision. In The Gambia, measurements on only one day each week, probably do not take sufficient account of daily or seasonal variations for precise estimates of an individual's intakes, but characteristic levels of intake could be demonstrated for clinical purposes. The response rate was virtually 100 per cent, as excellent co-operation was obtained in this community through the long-term residence of the investigators and the provision of medical care. Not all studies report such a high response rate.

6.3.4. Accuracy

In common with virtually all methods for the estimation of food intake, there is always concern that the results obtained may not be a reflection of usual food consumption. If the variety of foods eaten is limited and the meal pattern is constant it is unlikely that the food intake will alter on the measurement day. Serving food in a separate bowl, in The Gambia, introduced a degree of artificiality which was almost impossible to assess quantitatively. However, in that study it was believed to be as normal as possible from the mother's description and by the fieldworker's observations of the amounts of foods normally served in family food bowls. Another possible source of error is in the recall component for the between-meal foods, because subjects might under-report their consumption.

6.3.5. Validity

The observed weighed method has provided comparable within-community comparisons of food intake before and after a maternal dietary supplementation programme in The Gambia.[86] The results were also in accordance with the known agricultural availability of the different food crops and the highly seasonal nature of the food supply, and hence the energy and nutrient intake. The validity was tested using the doubly-labelled water technique.[88] Preliminary results indicated that the energy expenditure was higher than the energy intake as assessed by the observed weighed intake method.[97] More data are needed to explain this discrepancy between energy intake and expenditure.

When seasonal changes in body composition were taken into account, Norgan *et al.*[81] also found energy intakes in some groups of their Papua New Guinean subjects to be less than measured energy expenditure. Even so identical measurements made by them in a different village demonstrated excellent agreement between the two components. In their study, food intake was meticulously measured using the observed weighed intake record.

6.3.6. Precision

The purpose of the study determines the required precision of results. As described in 6.1.6. information about the within- and between-person variation is needed to calculate the required sample size and number of records needed for a specific degree of precision (14.1.3).

6.4. Records combined with direct chemical analysis

6.4.1. Principles

Samples for food analysis are necessary when accurate values in food composition tables are not available for the nutrient or food under investigation. The actual system adopted depends on the type of information required, the chemical methods used and the ingenuity of the investigators. There are, however, three general approaches:

● Food composites prepared after completion of the dietary survey. They consist of local foods and reflect the average daily food consumption as calculated from the records of intake.

● Complete duplicate collections of all foods immediately before consumption by the subject over a single day. This must be combined with a weighed dietary record survey because it is essential that each individual supplies an exact duplicate.

● The collection of small aliquots of each food eaten over the period of the survey by each individual immediately before consumption, the aliquots being placed in separate labelled containers.

6.4.2. Uses

Food composites are suitable for type 1 and type 2 information if estimates of the variance of food consumption are available from computer records. This approach has been used to estimate the intake of non-starch polysaccharides in Britain.[16] However, the method is not applicable where individual cooking and eating practices affect the results as, for example, in the measurement of vitamin C or resistant starch.

Complete duplicate collections are suitable for types 1 and 2 information with certain limitations and have been used to measure non-starch polysaccharide intake in Denmark and Finland.[53]

Duplicate collections, however, are not suitable for types 3 and 4 information where prolonged observations on individuals are necessary. This is because subjects do not supply accurate duplicates for longer than a single day.[61]

Aliquot technique is suitable in theory for all types of information (1–4) but it accumulates a great number of samples for chemical analysis. However, there is no alternative when individual information (types 3 and 4) on highly variable food constituents is required.

6.4.3. Practical aspects

Of the three approaches, the duplicate collection has most difficulty in gaining cooperation from subjects and hence accurate results. The subjects must be asked beforehand to buy sufficient food for an extra person and told that the cost will be refunded on the day of the collection. It must be emphasized that the duplicate collection will *not* be 'thrown away' or wasted. It is of crucial importance that a full collection of every morsel of food, including sugar in drinks, is obtained. This type of collection can only be undertaken when subjects have been taught how to weigh their food because there is evidence that unweighed duplicate collections of food are incomplete.[2] It is usual to plan for the duplicate collection on the final day of a survey, when subjects have become used to weighing their food.

Equipment

Pre-weighed rigid plastic containers of 2–3 litres capacity with lids are needed by each subject for duplicate portion collections. Pre-weighed screw-topped vials are used for aliquots. The type of container, amount of aliquot required and the preservative used for the food samples depends on the nutrient being investigated and must be decided on for the particular survey in question (6.1.2).

Instructions

The day before a planned duplicate portion collection, sample foods (e.g. breakfast cereal and sugar) should be used to demonstrate the food collection technique, and the subject should be asked to repeat the demonstration, using the instructions in Table 6.10.

If the subject normally eats all of his/her midday meals away from home, he/she should be asked to obtain a duplicate portion if possible

Table 6.10. Instructions for collecting duplicate food samples

1. It is essential that you collect, as duplicates, exactly the same foods as you eat on .... (give day and/or date). Please buy enough food to make meals for an extra person — you will be repaid for the cost of this extra food.

2. Check that you have a spare plate that is the same weight as the plate you use to eat from.

3. Weigh out the food to eat and record the details in the usual way. Keep it warm, if necessary.

4. On to the spare plate, weigh out exactly the same quantities of food in the same order as before. Put this duplicate meal to one side while you eat your meal.

5. After you have eaten your meal, weigh the leftovers in the usual way and remove exactly the same quantities from the duplicate meal on the spare plate.

6. Put the duplicate meal into the container.

7. You do not have to collect, but you must weigh and record as usual, the following:
   ● beer and all other alcoholic drinks
   ● soft drinks
   ● tea
   ● ground coffee
   ● water for instant coffee
   ● water and mineral water

8. On the collection day, a duplicate portion of ALL other foods eaten must be put into the container.
   This includes soup, sugar (including that used in drinks), cocoa powder, soft drink powders, and salt.

If you are unable to collect a duplicate portion of some foods please tell
M ....
Please keep your food containers in the refrigerator.

(for example, from snack bars or 'take-away' restaurants) for the midday meal. If this is not possible, the fieldworker will have to visit the place where the food was eaten and obtain a duplicate meal on that or the following day. If the subject normally has at least one midday meal at home, or takes a packed lunch, he/she should be asked to do this on the day of the duplicate collection to aid the procedure. The food container, and written instructions (Table 6.10) should be left with the subject.

A return visit should be made as early as possible on the day the subject is due to make the duplicate collection, to make a thorough check that the food is being weighed and collected, and the record kept. Repeat visits may be necessary during the day.

On the next day, the weighed food record (6.1) should be checked, ensuring that all the required information has been obtained. The field-worker should then calculate the total weight of food eaten, minus the weight of foods that need not be collected (Table 6.10) from the food record. The duplicate collection should then be weighed and compared with the calculated weight of the food recorded. If there is more than a 20 g difference the reason for the discrepancy must be found and corrected. If it is not possible to correct the discrepancy, an explanation must be written down on the food record. Before leaving, the fieldworker should make sure that the subject has been thanked and repaid for the cost of the food. The subject should be advised that if extra information is required about the food eaten, another visit or telephone call may be necessary.

Labelling and storage of food

The collected foods should be checked to see that there are no bones or stones in them, as these can damage homogenizing equipment. The treatment of the collection depends on the nutrient being investigated. If it is to be deep frozen care should be taken to double-wrap the collection with a typed label of the name, person number and date of collection on both the inner and outer wrappings.

It is not usual to collect the following drinks which have a high water content:

- beer and all other alcoholic drinks;
- soft drinks;
- tea;
- coffee;
- water for instant coffee;
- water and mineral water (Table 6.10).

6.4.4. Accuracy

Two factors affecting the accuracy of records combined with direct chemical analysis will be discussed in Chapter 8. Another factor more difficult to assess, is the completeness of the duplicates. In one study,[53] weights of food collected were compared with that reported. The chemically analysed contents of fat, carbohydrate, and nitrogen in the duplicate collections were compared with calculated intakes of the same day, using food composition tables and the food records. The overall correlation coefficients between protein intake calculated from the food tables and that in the duplicates, for example, was 0.86, slope 0.99, intercept 2.3 g protein. The standard deviations of individual percentage differences between analysed and calculated intakes of protein ranged from only 8 to 16 per cent in the four study areas, and those for fat from 7 to 21 per cent. Judged by this evidence, available from weighing and analysis, the food samples were thought to be virtually complete duplicates.[53]

6.5. Recall methods

The second category for collecting data about foods consumed is by interview. There are three methods: the 24-hour recall (this recalls the actual intake on a *specific* day); the dietary history (this assesses the *usual* intake over a period of time); and the food frequency (this assesses how often *specific foods* are eaten).

The main advantage of these recall methods is that they place minimal burdens on the subjects, compared with the dietary record methods already discussed. This is a crucial factor to consider when a high and non-biased cooperation rate in a survey must be obtained.

The main disadvantage of these methods is that the food consumption data collected is based entirely on the subjects' memory and judgement.

Apart from these common features the three methods are very different. Each has its own strengths and limitations and because of this they are suitable for different purposes. The following sections discuss their uses.

6.6. 24-hour recall (3.2.14)

6.6.1. Principle

By means of an interview the actual food intake of an individual is recalled for the immediate past 24 or 48 hours, or for the preceding day. For convenience the method is usually referred to as the '24-hour recall method' as this is the most common period to use. Food quantities are usually assessed by use of household measures, food models, or photographs. The method can be used to collect type 1 information.

This method was first mentioned by Burke in 1938 as a tool to teach mothers how to record the dietary intake of their child.[26] However, as the results were not calculated in terms of energy and nutrients, Wiehl, from her study of dietary deficiencies among industrial workers, is generally cited as being the first investigator to use this method.[117]

Recall methods have been used in many different ways. The length of time recalled has ranged from a few hours to 7 days, with 24 hours being the most common. Information may be obtained by the interviewer during a personal interview or by telephone, using either an open form, a precoded questionnaire, a tape-recorder, or a computer programme. As these different ways of collecting information may influence the study results, details on how the recall data were obtained should be explained clearly when the results are reported.

6.6.2. Practical aspects

Demands on the interviewer

The interviewer should be trained in the art of questioning and have a thorough knowledge of general food habits and commonly eaten foods in the study area and particularly among the target group. Subjects speaking a foreign language should be interviewed by an interpreter who must be familiar with their food habits. It is also important for the interviewer to have a thorough knowledge of the purpose of the study and the food composition table or data bank to be used during the subsequent data processing stage. This is important if enough relevant dietary detail is to be recalled in a form that is appropriate and can be coded.

During the interview the interviewer should keep an open mind and avoid showing signs of surprise, approval, or disapproval of the subject's diet (7.2.3).[125]

If more than one interviewer is involved in a study, a standardized protocol must be followed and the data obtained should be checked frequently to detect any systematic differences.

When using repeated recalls it may be an advantage to let the subject have the same interviewer each time throughout the study, though it is not essential. Well supervised studies following standardized procedures have not found any systematic interviewer effect.[10, 59]

Demands on the subjects

The recall method depends on the subject's ability to remember and adequately describe his/her diet. Thus it is not suitable for young children below the age of about 7 years, many old people above the age of 75 years or severely handicapped subjects if, for example, they are mentally impaired, blind, or have a speech problem. Obviously the demand on the memory is greater if the recall period is longer than 24 hours.

The method takes a minimum of time, approximately 15–20 minutes for a single 24-hour recall. No special skills, including writing, are needed by the subjects.

Recommended procedure

A well-conducted recall could follow the recommendations recently suggested by the Nordic Cooperation Group of Dietary Researchers:

1. Give no prior warning: the subjects should not know beforehand if or when they will be questioned about their food intake. Even though this could help memory of some subjects, others may change their usual diet in some way just for the occasion.

2. Always conduct the recall as an interview: a 24-hour recall may be personal or conducted by telephone. Though personal interviews are most common and probably provide the best interview situation, interviews by phone in areas where almost everybody has access to a private telephone, may save time and travel costs. However, in any study the mixing of these two approaches should be avoided as there is no written evidence that they provide data of similar quality. (N.B. It is not a 24-hour recall if a subject fills in a questionnaire concerning his consumption for a previous day.)

3. Location of interview: the interview should take place in a relaxed atmosphere in a quiet place. Since the location of the interview may influence the subject's ability and willingness to report his/her diet, all subjects within a study should be interviewed in the same type of place (7.2).

4. Even representation of days: ideally, the interviews should include recalls for all days of the week, especially if the study purpose is to describe the diet of particular groups of individuals. However, as this is not always possible, the distribution of recalls according to the days of the week and the season should be reported. An even representation of selected weekdays may suffice if dietary intakes of subgroups are to be compared or if results are to be compared before and after some kind of treatment, such as dietary advice.

5. Order of food recall: it is preferable to start with the first food/drink taken in the morning and proceed throughout the day. If any subjects are night workers their diet should be reported from midnight to midnight. Other starting points may be more appropriate if, in the study, people work odd hours. When more than 24 hours are to be recalled, they should start with the most recent food intake and work backwards. However, little is known about the feasibility and completeness of such extended recalls.

6. Use of neutral questions: the interviewer should use neutral questions like '*when?*' and '*what* did you eat or drink ... after you woke up in the morning, before you left home, on your way to work or school, at work or school?', or simply '*what* did you have the next?' No question should be suggestive or lead the subject to an answer. To be able to ask good questions requires detailed knowlege of local foods, general activities, and ways of eating among the particular group being studied. Usual food combinations may not be explained during the interview unless the interviewer knows about them and specifically asks 'Did you have anything on, in or with it, for example, butter or margarine on

bread, sugar or milk in tea or on ceral, ketchup with the hot dog?' Details like brand names, the physical nature of the food item and, if homemade, the method of preparation, may be asked for, according to the purpose of the study. A standard list, picture, or photograph of snack foods commonly used by the target group may be presented at the end of the interview, as an aid to memory.[44]

7. Estimation of amounts: graduated food models of some sort (7.1.3) are highly recommended, as well as a selection of familiar household cups, glasses, bowls, and spoons for estimating food quantity. A ruler may also be of help to determine the size of other types of foods. If food models are used they should not be shown until needed for quantifying specific foods. A picture book, a selection of natural foods, or realistic food models may be presented at the close of the interview as an additional memory aid. If the subject eats one or more meals in a school or company canteen, average serving sizes may be determined by the investigators for the relevant days. If phone interviews are to be used a booklet with pictures or drawings of food servings may be sent to the subject before the interview takes place.

8. Open-ended form: names of meals or foods or codes for foods or food amounts may be provided on the form to aid writing during the interview. If the recall is to be conducted through a computer programme the questions asked should be designed to be neutral as possible.

6.6.3. Uses, examples, and limitations

The 24-hour recall method has several practical advantages. It is quick and simple to perform, places a minimal burden on the subject and is applicable to most target groups regardless of their background. Field costs are relatively low and the response rates are high compared with other methods already described. For these reasons, the recall methods have been especially attractive to use in large field studies where a representative sample is particularly important, as in the Nutrition Canada National Survey[82] and HANES I and II.[122]

Two major disadvantages of the method should be kept in mind. There is a problem with memory and food descriptions, but this may be minimized by a carefully conducted standardized interview procedure. A more serious problem is the large intra-individual or day-to-day variation found in many groups, especially in industrialized countries. For this reason a single 24-hour recall should only be used in studies examining the mean level of food and nutrient intake of a group (type 1 information). For other types of information repeated 24-hour recalls are necessary.

The 24-hour recall may be used to describe the diet of selected groups in order to find evidence of any potential dietary problem in the locality. This would be used to form the basis of educational programmes. However, as recall studies often do not include Fridays, Saturdays, or Sundays, the group average may not be a true picture of the group food consumption.

The method may also be used as a component of a dietary history in clinical or epidemiological studies and as a way of teaching about the desirable details to be recorded in a dietary history record form.

Use of repeated recalls

Provided that a sufficient number of repetitions are done, repeated recalls may be an alternative method to use in studies requiring group means and distribution (type 2 information) or classification of individuals according to distributions of intake (type 3 information). If the usual intake of people with irregular meal patterns and food habits are to be studied, repeated recalls may be the most appropriate method to use.

In studies using repeated recalls a drop out of subjects should be anticipated. This is because either they cannot be reached on a planned interview date or they no longer fulfil the criteria for being in the study.[33] Once recruited, only a few subjects seem to withdraw because of an unwillingness to co-operate.[10, 103] Unless they are done by telephone, costs for repeated recalls will be higher than for a single one (7.2.3). It might be cheaper to let the subjects recall several consecutive days rather than arrange for separate interview sessions. However, as stated earlier extended recalls may only be feasible with very special groups.[4, 43, 92]

6.6.4. Validity

In institution and canteen settings it is possible to observe and measure the actual intake without the awareness of the subject and thus do a direct validation of the recalled intake. Studies in which this has been done are summarized in review articles.[7,24,91] Several of the studies report acceptable group means while others have found that the recall method underestimates the actual intake.

The somewhat contradictory results on the group level may be due to differences in the study design, how the quantities have been estimated and the results have been expressed. In addition different population groups may show varying results. Women tend to give more accurate information about their diet than men, in validation studies of different age and sex groups, and middle-aged subjects the best results.[32, 59] So far, no one has been able to do a direct validation study on the total diet of people living in their own homes.

Comparison with other methods

A number of studies have measured the relative validity of the 24-hour recall by comparing it with another method. For group means, the method shows good agreement with estimated and weighed food records, even though a few studies have come to other conclusions.[7, 24, 91]

The recall tends to provide lower group means and larger variance than the dietary history. Large discrepancies are more common between dietary history and the 24-hour recall method than between weighed or estimated food records and the 24-hour recall. The ability of the methods to produce comparable estimates varies greatly with the food or nutrient under consideration.[7]

6.6.5. Precision

The precision of reproducibility of group means may be improved by repeating the recalls and increased sample size will do the same. According to Beaton *et al.*[10] it would be preferable in most cases to use a single interview with an increased sample size rather than repeating the recalls (type 1 information). However, when the analysis and interpretation of the data is to go further than to group means, repeated interviews are strongly recommended, at least on sub-samples.

The number of repeated recalls necessary to obtain a reasonable precision in classifying individuals' intakes for food groups and nutrients depends upon the nutrient in question and the food pattern of the specific population group. The same factors have been described for record methods in 6.1.6.

Repeated recalls may provide an acceptable classification of individual intakes for food groups and nutrients that show a low to moderate variability. If the daily variation is extreme, as it often can be, when dietary cholestrol or vitamin A are involved, an acceptable classification may not be obtained unless many recalls are taken (Table 6.5 and 6.6).

Improved correlations between nutrient intake and indicators of nutritional status have been demonstrated for repeated recalls when compared with single-day recalls.[101]

6.7. Dietary history (3.2.15)

6.7.1. Principle

The dietary history method assesses an individual's total food intake and usual meal pattern over varying periods of time. In theory, it may refer to any given period of the past, but more usually to the last month, last 6 months, or the last year. The information is best obtained by a nutritionist, or someone with relevant training in the food and nutrition field, during a personal interview. The dietary history might be used for types 2 and 3 information, but it is not efficient for type 1. The method for a dietary history must fulfil the following criteria:

● assess the total food intake;

● include information on the usual meal pattern and food combinations separate from the dietary information obtained by a check list of foods;

● estimate portion sizes.

Burke and her co-workers[27] developed the dietary history technique in three parts. The first was an interview about the subject's usual pattern of intake with the food quantities specified in household measures. The second was a cross-check using a detailed list of foods to verify and clarify the overall eating pattern. Finally, the subject recorded her food intake at home, in household measures, for 3 days.

Today the original method is seldom used. It has been changed by other investigators[9] and the 3-day food record is usually left out. Although their method is very different from the original one, some investigators still claim to have used 'the Burke method'.

6.7.2. Practical aspects

In an open interview, firmly controlled by the interviewer, the subject is questioned about a typical day's eating pattern. Alternatively, the interview may start with a 24-hour recall.

Each meal is discussed in turn to find out which foods were used and how often, what alternatives might be used on other days of the week and any irregularities in the eating pattern, so that a menu can be established for 7 days or for a month.

Usual portion sizes are estimated with the aid of food models or replicas (8.1.3) and given information can be cross-checked using a list of individual foods as a memory aid.

As for the 24-hour recall, the purpose of the study must be so well known that it is easy for the interviewer to judge what information must be collected. A carefully prepared form is often used to record information and the interview lasts about 1–1.5 hours.

In a collaborative study all interviewers must have followed the same protocol for training and be visited at regular intervals during field work. Frequent checks should be made to detect any systematic differences between interviewers.

It would be very difficult for a non-nutritionist to carry out a dietary history interview unless it was firmly guided and controlled by a specially made, precoded interview form.

As discussed in 7.2.3, demands are made of the interviewer, but they are also made on the subject. These include an assumption that memory and an ability to make judgements will neither consciously nor sub-consciously distort the information report. Because the dietary history is more abstract than a 24-hour recall, it is a more demanding interview for the subject. Consequently it is not usual to obtain a satisfactory history from children less than 14 years old or from the elderly over 80 years of age, though maturity and mental state cannot be set by any fixed age.[71]

Two alternatives to the open interview have been suggested for obtaining a dietary history. One uses a pre-coded interview form (6.2.2), but though it might have possibilities for non-nutritionist professional interviewers, it almost doubles the interview time.[63] The other alternative, said to be closely related to a dietary history, is the use of self-administered food-use-questionnaires.[31, 85] However, as these provide very limited information about meal patterns, it is difficult for this type of questionnaire to fulfil the criteria demanded for the dietary history.

6.7.3. Uses, examples, and limitations

The dietary history method has two main advantages. First, it gives information on the diet over a long period of time. Second, it requires limited effort by the subjects so that high cooperation rates can be achieved in surveys.

The major disadvantage of the method is that it has a high subjective component because the information it collects is based entirely on an individual's memory and report. Another disadvantage is that the method concentrates on the regular patterns so that irregularities are easily underestimated.

As already stated a dietary history may cover any given period of the past, but the maximal time period possible is debatable. Probably it is not realistic to try to cover a whole year, although some investigators do. This is particularly relevant for foods that show strong seasonal fluctuation because the dietary history answers are likely to be strongly influenced by the immediate past.[20] In any study it is important to specify how long a period the dietary history should cover.

Information on the pattern of meals is found by a dietary history, but the regularity of the pattern may be exaggerated. The history provides data on the consumption of individual foods and is able to focus on specific foods, but information on day-to-day variation in food or nutrient intake cannot be obtained by this method. As the dietary history covers the total diet, energy and nutrient intakes can be calculated.

The method can be used to assess the *relative* average intakes of groups of people and the distribution of the intakes in the group, but there is some doubt about its suitability for assessing the average of *absolute* intakes of the group. Data collected by this method can be used to rank individuals relatively and to classify them into broad categories according to their intake, but it should not be used to assess the absolute intake of individuals. A dietary history, therefore, is not an adequate method if absolute nutrient intake is to be directly related to clinical, biochemical, or other measurements on an individual basis.

Burke recommended that her method should be used only for rating the intake (for example as 'excellent' or 'poor' when compared with recommended intakes). She said, 'using exact figures gives an unjustified impression of the accuracy of the data'.[27]

The dietary history is unsuitable for collecting data from subjects who have no regular pattern of eating. Neither is it suitable for a survey which has a focus on foods which are typical of irregular or impulse eating such as alcohol, sweets, and so on.

6.7.4. Validity

The validity of a dietary history depends both on the subject's ability to give correct information on frequencies and an ability to estimate portion sizes correctly. Furthermore, validity can be markedly influenced by the food models or other aids used in the study.

The dietary history's validity can only be measured relative to another method. For example, it can be compared with the recording of food intake in a prospective study. However, the recording must cover a sufficiently long period to allow individual comparisons of the two methods. Pietinen *et al.*,[85] when validating their method, used twelve 2-day food records over a period of 6 months. Reported validation studies seldom cover a sufficiently long period.

On the individual level, assessment of the *absolute* energy and nutrient intake by dietary history and by a 7-day food record gives different results. Obviously the two methods do not measure the same thing. At the group level, the mean nutrient intakes assessed by the dietary history are often higher than when assessed by either measured or weighed food records. However, this result is not consistent and other investigators have found similar or lower mean nutrient intakes when comparing the dietary history with food records.[20,56,71,85]

The *relative* intakes assessed by the two methods seem to be more consistent. When individuals are ranked and then classified in thirds according to their energy intake, half to one-third of the subjects are usually placed in the same class by both methods, but 5–10 per cent may be grossly misclassified by being placed in the opposite thirds.[20,24,71] How these misclassifications reduce the value of the relative risk estimates in epidemiological studies has been explained by Marshall *et al.*[74] and Walker and Blettner.[112] Though it is beyond the scope of this book to explain these statistical problems, it should be kept in mind that reducing the relative risk estimates has important implications for sample size requirements.

6.7.5. Precision

Studies on the precision or reproducibility of dietary histories show fairly good agreement for energy, protein, fat, and carbohydrate for up to 2 years, but the reproducibility for other nutrients is variable and sometimes poor.[8,24,49,71,85,100,108]

Reproducibility depends heavily upon the target group, the time of reference and on the foods and nutrients of interest. Another important aspect is the time interval between the two estimates. This depends on the time of reference of the method. For example, if the time of reference is the usual food consumption in a specific season, all estimates have to be done within that season. The most desirable time interval is a dilemma because any influence on the second estimate by the first one should be avoided. One influence could be, for example, due to a recollection of the first interview and yet, the longer the time interval, the greater the probability that food habits will change.

In general, the reproducibility of the dietary history is better than for the 24-hour recall or the 24-hour estimated or weighed record, because results of a dietary history method do not take into account the day-to-day variation.

6.7.6. Final comments

Before planning to use the dietary history it is necessary to evaluate critically if the characteristics of the diet, important for the study, can be measured properly by a method with a strong subjective component and one which focuses on the regular part of the diet.

A detailed description of the method should always be included when results are reported. It should include information such as: the length of the interview, the training of the interviewers, the estimation of portion sizes, the validity and the precision of the method in that particular study.

The term 'dietary history' should only be used if the method fulfils the definition presented in 3.2.15 and at the beginning of this section.

6.8. Food frequency (3.2.16)

6.8.1. Principle

The food frequency method estimates how frequently certain foods are eaten during a specified period of time.

One of the drawbacks of the methods described so far in this chapter is that they are time consuming, require much training on the part of the investigator and cooperation on the part of the subject. The 24-hour recalls are valid for group values (type 1 information), but not for classifying subjects into high, medium, or low consumers of certain foods and/or nutrients (type 3 information). Faced with these problems a number of investigators have attempted to develop a method which is valid, but cheaper and easier to apply in epidemiological studies. The most common approach is the food frequency method, originally outlined as a short schedule for qualitative classification of dietary patterns.[118]

The first questionnaires developed would not include quantitative estimates other than as so many servings or portions per day/week/month. The data produced is based on the assumption that portion size does not vary to any great extent, at least for a given study group. This is a gross assumption and therefore some investigators have built into the technique a quantitative aspect to try to overcome this problem.

There are two approaches possible in using a food frequency method. One depends on a record with communication through the mail, while the other conducts a short interview. Both approaches may, or may not, include quantitative assessments.

To estimate nutrient intake, food frequency scores for individual items are multiplied by the nutrient content of the local standard portion or estimated portion size.

Depending on the purpose of the study, information is sought only on those foods or nutrients which are relevant to the aim(s) of the study.

6.8.2. Practical aspects

The design of the food frequency questionnaire or interview usually requires more time from the investigator than questionnaires concerning the 24-hour recall or dietary history methods.

In developing the questionnaire the investigator should answer the following questions:

1. How many and which food items are necessary to give sufficient information on the dietary component of interest? A good questionnaire enables the investigator to classify subjects as small, medium, or large consumers. Only those foods that contribute to the variance of dietary components of interest should be included in the questionnaire. It is possible to determine this variance from large scale surveys which have already examined the food consumption in great detail.[120]

2. Are the instructions to the questionnaire sufficiently clear for completion by the respondent or non-technical personnel?

3. Is it possible for the respondent to give correct estimates of frequency, especially for seasonal foods, and, if necessary, of portion sizes?
4. How many open ended questions will be included in the questionnaire? These questions may extend the accuracy but increase the need for manual coding.
5. How many qualitative questions should be included to account for the effects of using, during food preparation, fat, sugar, salt, and/or other dietary components of interest for the study?
6. How many additional questions that may be relevant for the purpose of the study should be incorporated?

Food frequency questionnaires in general are developed for specific purposes and specific population groups. If an investigator wants to use an existing questionnaire for another purpose and/or population group, this questionnaire should first be validated. Figure 14.3 gives an example of a food frequency questionnaire.

6.8.3. Examples, uses, and limitations

The food frequency method has been used in several studies investigating possible associations between diet and health,[19,29,46,90,120] to evaluate nutrition education programmes,[63] and to examine dietary compliance.

The *advantages* of the food frequency are that it is a cheap, simple, quick method which can be completed by the subjects themselves or personnel without special training. Most questionnaires are pre-coded which makes collected data simple to treat.

The *disadvantage* of the method is that the development of the questionnaire is difficult and tedious work.

Data collected with the questionnaire is rather limited and for most questionnaires excludes the possibility of analysing the data in relation to other dietary components, about which questions were not asked.

6.8.4. Validity

A number of authors have compared the food frequency method with the dietary history method and with the estimated or weighed record methods.[5,28,34,41,105] Some questionnaires have given better results than others. The relative validity of food frequency questionnaires estimating a limited number of dietary components is, in general, better than the relative validity of the food frequency questionnaires trying to estimate total diet.

Some investigators[3,48,50] have tried to make use of prediction equations to permit quantification on the basis of short questionnaires. These studies have involved considerable effort, questionnable generalizations and a disappointing level of prediction.

6.8.5. Precision

Very few studies have examined the precision or reproducibility of food frequency questionnaires. As for dietary histories, the problem for such an evaluation is the time interval between the test and re-test. In two studies[28,80] the agreement found between test and re-test varied between nutrients, but, in general, was not very high.

6.8.6. Final comments

Methods involving food frequencies or other types of short questionnaire seem to be very attractive for epidemiological studies. However, the information collected is limited and the development of the question-naire requires a great deal of effort from the investigator.

Unfortunately this type of questionnaire is often used where it is not appropriate, such as in studies interested in estimating the level of energy intake of a specific group.

6.9. Retrospective dietary assessments

6.9.1. Principle

Retrospective dietary assessments use the dietary history and/or food frequency methods to assess the intake in the distant past, which may be many years ago. There are several procedures to follow. Usually subjects are questioned about their current diet in order to establish a base line to which retrospective information can be linked. Before starting with the retrospective assessment special questions are added to the dietary history or food frequency to help the subject remember his/her food habits in the distant past during the period of interest for the study.

6.9.2. Practical aspects

The practical aspects described for the dietary history and/or food frequency methods should be taken into account when using either of these methods for retrospective dietary assessments. The method to be used depends on the purpose of the epidemiological study. A subject's current dietary habits are closely related to what is recalled about the past and they should be carefully scrutinized. Specific questions about the individual's changes in habits and about preferences should be asked. A dietary history exploring and assessing past food habits is not easy and the interview takes time. Interview training to become familiar with the questionnaire and its aims is of great importance.

For the current, as well as the retrospective assessment, the time of reference should be clearly pointed out.

6.9.3. Uses, examples, and limitations

Methods assessing past dietary habits have been developed for use in case-control studies examining exposure to food factors thought to be of importance in the aetiology of a disease.

However, in making comparisons between patients and healthy controls, it is not known whether the measured risk factor is a cause or effect of the disease in question. In the study of diet this is particularly true. The most common symptoms in gastrointestinal disease are pain and altered bowel function[36] which the patient may attempt to improve by a change in diet. Almost always a person's diet is a mixture of nutrients and other components, all of which can cause a variety of endogenous reactions, interactions, and other effects. Thus a dietary factor carrying a high risk may, in the presence of others, be rendered harmless. Consequently the aim of dietary investigations in most case-control studies is to find out the combinations of foods eaten in the past and before the onset of symptoms.

Retrospective dietary assessments have further limitations in addition to those already described in sections 6.7 and 6.8 about the dietary history and food frequency methods. These must also be taken into account:

1. Subjects find it hard to remember past dietary habits and more specifically combinations of foods taken during one meal.

2. Current dietary habits influence the recall of past dietary habits.[59,102]

3. Estimating portion sizes used in the past is difficult. Only approximations of nutrient intakes can be made.

6.9.4. Accuracy

A number of studies in various countries have been made to assess the relative validity of retrospective assessments.[28,45,55,57,64,93,102] The subjects in the studies were people who had participated in food consumption studies in the past. Data of these initial food consumption studies were taken as the reference and data from recent retrospective dietary interviews were compared with it.

Most studies discuss their findings in the light of the requirements of a case-control study where the relative placing of participants into categories is of primary importance. The information collected in these studies provides empirical data about the possible degree of misclassification in such studies. Misclassification can influence the conclusions of the study considerably.[23,75,112,113]

A specific problem in this method is the observed effect of current food intake on the recall of past diet. Validation studies carried out so far have been conducted with healthy subjects. If cancer patients who may have changed their diet as a result of disease and treatment are also influenced by their current intake, their recall of past food intake is probably affected more than has been found for healthy subjects. This fact might lead to differential misclassifications in case-control studies.

Until now there has been no agreement on how much misclassification is acceptable for a study and there is little knowledge on the degree of differential misclassifications among those with disease and the healthy controls. A case-control study within a prospective study may give more information on these problems.[110]

6.9.5. Final comments

There is little experience, so far, in the use of retrospective assessments. Investigators wanting to use these methods in case-control studies should pre-test their questionnaire. A good design of the case-control study may be helpful in conducting the food consumption study. In summary, the problems of examining the role of food factors in the aetiology of the disease are:

(1) the determination of the time frame for the food consumption study;

(2) the conduct of the study before the patients feel themselves seriously ill;

(3) the difficulty in helping the respondents to recall their food consumption from the distant past and to remember the combinations of foods they used to have in meals.

6.10. Combined methods

There is no best method for all study purposes. As has been described in the various sections of this chapter each method has specific advantages and disadvantages.

Table 6.11 summarizes the main sources of error and variation associated with five of the methods of estimating food consumption.[13,98,99]

These sources of error and variation make a method more, or less useful for the type of information needed.

Table 6.12 summarizes the possible approaches there are for the different types of information.[11]

Table 6.11. Sources of error in methods estimating food consumption

Sources of error	Duplicate portion	Weighed record	Estimated record	24-h recall	Dietary history
Response errors					
omitting foods	−	±	±	+	+
adding foods	−	−	−	+	+
estimation of weight of foods	−	−	+	+	+
estimating frequency of consumption of foods	−	−	−	−	+
day to day variation	+	+	+	+	−
changes in diet	+	+	±	−	−
Coding errors	−	+	+	+	+
Errors in conversion into nutrients					
food composition tables	−	+	+	+	+
sampling errors	+	−	−	−	−
direct analysis	+	−	−	−	−

+ error is likely.
− error is unlikely.

Table 6.12. Possible approaches for different types of information

Type of information	Possible approach
Mean food consumption of a group	Single weighed/estimated food record, single 24-hour recall
Mean and distribution of food consumption in a group	Repeated weighed/estimated food record, repeated 24-hour recall, dietary history
Relative magnitude of the food consumption of an individual as belonging to a certain third or fifth of the distribution of intakes	Multiple repeated weighed/estimated food record, multiple repeated 24-hour recall, dietary history
The absolute magnitude of the usual food consumption of an individual	This is a problem (Table 6.5)

A combination of two methods might give more information or might make a study easier to carry out. Combined methods have, in fact, already been described in several sections of this chapter:

- 6.1.1. a weighed record with estimations of foods eaten in restaurants;
- 6.3.2. an observed weighed record combined with a recall of foods eaten between meals;

• 6.7.2. a 24-hour food recall incorporated in a dietary history method.

Sometimes in national food consumption surveys a combination is used of a household food record and a 24-hour food recall of individuals within the household. The application of the 24-hour food recall may be limited, for example, to individuals within a vulnerable age group. A combination of methods can give information on food purchases and the availability of foods in different categories of households, on methods of food preparation, and on the mean food intake of one or more vulnerable categories of individuals.

If an investigator decides to use such a combination of methods, the whole procedure should be carefully pre-tested (Chapter 14), as the procedure might become a very heavy burden for the housekeeper.

References

1. Abakada, A. O. and Hussain, M. A. (1980). Nutritional status and dietary intake of lactating Yoruba mothers in Nigeria. *Ecol. Food Nutr.* **10**, 105–11.
2. Abdulla, M., Andersson, I., Asp, N. G., *et al.* (1981). Nutrient intake and health status of vegetarians. Chemical analysis of diets using the duplicate portion sampling technique. *Am. J. Clin. Nutr.* **34**, 2464–77.
3. Abramson, J. H., Slome, C., and Kosovsky, C. (1963). Food frequency interview as an epidemiological tool. *Am. J. Publ. Hlth* **53**, 1093–1101.
4. Adelson, S. F. (1960). Some problems in collecting dietary data from individuals. *J. Am. Diet Assoc.* **36**, 453–61.
5. Balogh, M., Kahn, H. A., and Medalie, J. H. (1971). Random repeat 24-hour dietary recalls. *Am. J. Clin. Nutr.* **24**, 304–10.
6. Barasi, M. E., Philips, K. M., and Burr, M. L. (1985). A weighed survey of women in South Wales. *Hum. Nutr. Appl. Nutr.* **39A**, 189–94.
7. Bazzarre, T. and Myers, M. (1978). The collection of food intake data in cancer epidemiology studies. *Nutr. Cancer* **1**, 22–45.
8. Bazzarre, T. L. and Yuhas, A. (1983). Comparative evaluation of methods of collecting food intake data for cancer epidemiology studies. *Nutr. Cancer* **5**, 201–14.
9. Beal, V. A. (1967). The nutritional history in longitudinal research. *J. Am. Diet Assoc.* **51**, 426–32.
10. Beaton, G. H., Milner, J., Corey, P., *et al.* (1979). Sources of variance in 24-hour dietary recall data: implications for nutrition study design and interpretation. *Am. J. Clin. Nutr.* **32**, 2546–59.
11. Beaton, G. H. (1982). What do we think we are measuring. In: *Symposium on dietary data collection analysis and significance.* Research Bulletin No. 675, Boston University of Massachusetts.
12. Bingham, S., McNeil, N. I., and Cummings, J. H. (1981). The diet of individuals: a study of a randomly chosen cross section of British adults in a Cambridgeshire village. *Br. J. Nutr.* **45**, 23–25.
13. Bingham, S., Wiggins, H. S., Englyst, H., *et al.* (1982). Methods and validity

of dietary assessments in four Scandinavian populations. *Nutr. Cancer* **4**, 23–33.

14. Bingham, S. (1983). Premise and methods. In: *Surveillance of the dietary habits of the population with regard to cardiovascular diseases.* (Backer, G. G. de, Tunstall, P. H., Pedoe, H., and Ducimetière, P., eds). EURO-NUT Report 2, Wageningen.

15. Bingham, S. and Cummings, J. H. (1983). The use of 4-amino benzoic acid as a marker to validate the completeness of 24-h urine collections in man. *Clin. Sci.* **64**, 629–35.

16. Bingham, S. A., Williams, D. R. R., and Cummings, J. H. (1985). Dietary fibre consumption in Britain: new estimates and their relation to large bowel cancer mortality. *Br. J. Cancer* **52**, 399–402.

17. Bingham, S. and Cummings, J. H. (1985). Urine nitrogen as an independent validatory measure of dietary intake. *Am. J. Clin. Nutr.* **42**, 1276–89.

18. Bingham, S. (1987). The dietary assessment of individuals; methods, accuracy, new techniques, and recommendations. *Nutr. Abs. Rev.* (in press).

19. Bjelke, E. (1975). Dietary vitamin A and human lung cancer. *Intl. J. Cancer* **15**, 561–5.

20. Black, A. E. (1981). Pitfall in dietary assessment. In: *Recent advances in clinical nutrition.* (Howard, A. N. and McLean Baird, I., eds) pp. 11–18. John Libbey, London.

21. Black, A. E., Cole, T. J., Wiles, S. J., and White, F. (1983). Daily variation in food intake of infants from 2 to 18 months. *Hum. Nutr. Appl. Nutr.* **37A**, 448–58.

22. Black, A. E., Ravenscroft, C., and Sims, A. J. (1984). The NACNE Report: are dietary goals realistic? Comparisons with the dietary patterns of dietitians. *Hum. Nutr. Appl. Nutr.* **38A**, 165–79.

23. Blettner, M. and Wahrendorf, J. (1984). What does an observed relative risk convey about possible misclassification. *Methods Inf. Med.* **23**, 37–40.

24. Block, G. (1982). A review of validations of dietary assessment methods. *Am. J. Epidemiol.* **115**, 492–505.

25. Bransby, E. R., Daubney, C. G., and King, J. (1948). Comparison of results obtained by different methods of individual dietary survey. *Br. J. Nutr.* **2**, 89–110.

26. Burke, B. S. and Stuart, H. C. (1938). A method of diet analysis. Application in research and pediatrics practice. *J. Pediat.* **12**, 493–503.

27. Burke, B. S. (1947). The dietary history as a tool in research. *J. Am. Diet Assoc.* **23**, 1041–6.

28. Byers, T. E., Rosenthal, R. T., Marshall, J. R., Rzepka, T. F., Cummings, M., and Graham, S. (1983). Dietary history from the distant past: a methodological study. *Nutr. Cancer* **5**, 69–77.

29. Byers, T. E. (1984). The case-control study as a tool for studying the relationship between nutrition and cancer. In: *European collaborative study on the role of diet and other factors in the aetiology of atrophic gastritis: a precancerous lesion of gastric cancer.* (West, C. E., ed.). EURO-NUT Report 4. Wageningen.

30. Callmer, E., Hagman, U., Haraldsdóttir, J., Løken, E. B., Seppänen, R., and Trygg, K. (1986). Proposal for the standardisation of 24-hour recall and

similar interview methods. *Vår Föda* **38** (suppl 4), 259–68.
31. Callmer, E. (1987). (Personal communication.)
32. Campbell, V. A. and Dodds, M. L. (1967). Collecting dietary information from groups of older people. *J. Am. Diet Assoc.* **51**, 29–33.
33. Chappell, G. M. (1955). Long term individual dietary surveys. *Br. J. Nutr.* **9**, 323–39.
34. Chu, S. Y., Kolonel, L. N., Hankin, J. H., and Lee, J. (1984). A comparison of frequency and quantitative dietary methods for epidemiologic studies of diet and disease. *Am. J. Epidemiol.* **119**, 323–34.
35. Cole, T. and Black, A. (1984). Statistical aspects in the design of dietary surveys. In: *MRC Report No. 4.* Environmental Epidemiology Unit Southampton.
36. Cummings, J. H. (1981). Dietary fibre and large bowel cancer. *Proc. Nutr. Soc.* **40**, 7–14.
37. Darke, S. J., Disselduff, M. M., and Try, G. P. (1980). Frequency distribution of mean intakes of food energy and selected nutrients during nutrition surveys of different groups of people in Great Britain between 1968 and 1971. *Br. J. Nutr.* **44**, 243–52.
38. Ducimetière, P. (1983). Data analysis problems. In: *Surveillance of the dietary habits in the population with regard to cardiovascular diseases.* EURO-NUT Report 2, pp. 81–92. Wageningen.
39. Emmons, L. and Hayes, M. (1973). Accuracy of 24-hour recalls of young children. *J. Am. Diet Assoc.* **62**, 409–15.
40. Eppright, E. S., Patton, M. B., Marlatt, A. L., and Hathaway, M. L. (1952). Dietary study methods. V. Some problems in collecting dietary information about groups of children. *J. Am. Diet Assoc.* **28**, 43–8.
41. Epstein, L. M., Reshef, A., Abramson, J. H., and Bialik, O. (1970). Validity of a short dietary questionnaire. *Israel J. Med. Sci.* **6**, 589–97.
42. Fehilly, A. M., Phillips, K. M., and Sweetnam, P. M. (1984). A weighed dietary survey of men in Caerphilly, South Wales. *Hum. Nutr. Appl. Nutr.* **38A**, 270–6.
43. Flores, M., Flores, Z., and Lara, M. Y. (1965). Estimation of family and mother's dietary intake comparing two methods. *Trop. Geogr. Med.* **17**, 135–45.
44. Frank, G. C., Berenson, G. S., Schilling, P. E., and Moore, M. C. (1977). Adapting the 24-hr recall for epidemiologic studies of school children. *J. Am. Diet Assoc.* **71**, 26–31.
45. Garland, B., Ibrahim, M., and Grimson, R. (1982). Assessment of past diet in cancer epidemiology. *Am. J. Epidemiol.* **166**, 577 (abstract).
46. Haenszel, W., Kurihara, M., Segi, M., and Lee, R. K. C. (1972). Stomach cancer among Japanese in Hawaii. *JNCI* **49**, 969–88.
47. Hackett, A. F., Rugg-Gunn, A. J., and Appleton, D. R. (1983). Use of a dietary diary and interview to estimate the food intake of children. *Hum. Nutr. Appl. Nutr.* **37A**, 293–300.
48. Hankin, J. H., Rawlings, V., and Nomura, A. (1978). Assessment of a short dietary method for a prospective study on cancer. *Am. J. Clin. Nutr.* **31**, 355–9.
49. Hankin, J. H., Nomura, A. M. J., Lee, J., Hirohata, T., and Kolonel, L. N.

(1983). Reproducibility of a diet history questionnaire in a case-control study of breast cancer. *Am. J. Clin. Nutr.* **37**, 981–5.

50. Heady, J. A. (1961). Diets of bank clerks: development of a method of classifying the diets of individuals for use in epidemiological studies. *J. R. Stat. Soc.* **124**, 336–71.

51. Heslov, I. B. and Elsborg, L. (1976). Nutritional studies on long term surgical patients with special reference to the intake of vitamin B_{12} and folic acid. *Intl. J. Vit. Nutr. Res.* **46**, 427–32.

52. Huenemann, R. L. and Turner, D. (1942). Methods of dietary investigation. *J. Am. Diet Assoc.* **18**, 562–8.

53. IARC Large Bowel Cancer Group (1982). Second IARC international collaborative study on diet and large bowel cancer in Denmark and Finland. *Nutr. Cancer* **4**, 3–79.

54. Isaksson, B. (1980). Urinary nitrogen output as a validity test in dietary surveys. *Am. J. Clin. Nutr.* **33**, 4–5.

55. Jain, M., Howe, G. R., Johnson, K. C., and Miver, A. B. (1980). Evaluation of a diet history questionnaire for epidemiological studies. *Am. J. Epidemiol.* **111**, 212–19.

56. James, W. P. T., Bingham, S. A., and Cole, T. J. (1981). Epidemiological assessment of dietary intake. *Nutr. Cancer* **2**, 203–12.

57. Jensen, O. M., Wahrendorf, J., Rosenquist, A., and Geser, A. (1984). The reliability of questionnaire-derived historic dietary information and temporal stability of food habits in individuals. *Am. J. Epidemiol.* **120**, 281–90.

58. Johnson, N. E., Sempos, C. T., Elmer, P. J., Allington, J. K., and Matthews, M. E. (1982). Development of a dietary intake monitoring system for nursing homes. *J. Am. Diet Assoc.* **80**, 549–57.

59. Karvetti, R-L. and Knuts, L-R. (1985). Validity of 24-hour recall. *J. Am. Diet Assoc.* **85**, 1437–42.

60. Keys, A. (1970). Coronary heart disease in seven countries. *Circulation* (suppl. 1) **XLI** and **XLII**, 162–98.

61. Kim, W. W., Mertz, W., Judd, J. T., *et al.* (1984). Effect of making duplicate food collections on nutrient intakes calculated from diet records. *Am. J. Clin. Nutr.* **40**, 1333–7.

62. Kok, F. J., Matroos, A. W., Hautvast, J. G. A. J., and Ban, A. W. van den (1982). Food consumption pattern of the Dutch population in 1978, application of a qualitative history recall method. *Voeding* **43**, 14–23.

63. Larsen, P. H. L., Jensen, J. H., and Haraldsdóttir, J. (1985). The dietary history method with professional interviews and a precoded questionnaire. (Abstr.) Presented at 13th International Congress of Nutrition, Brighton, England.

64. Leeuwen, F. E. van, Vet, H. C. W. de, Hayes, R. B., *et al.* (1983). An assessment of the relative validity of retrospective interviewing for measuring dietary intake. *Am. J. Epidemiol.* **118**, 752–8.

65. Liu, K., Stamler, J., Dyer, A., McKeever, J., and McKeever, P. (1978). Statistical methods to assess and minimize the role of intra-individual variability in obscuring the relationship between dietary lipids and serum cholesterol. *J. Chron. Dis.* **31**, 399–418.

66. Logan, R. L., Thomson, M., Riemersma, R. A., *et al.* (1978). Risk factors for ischaemic heart disease in normal men aged 40. *Lancet* **i**, 949–55.
67. Madden, J. P., Goodman, S. J., and Guthrie, H. A. (1976). Validity of the 24-hour recall. *J. Am. Diet Assoc.* **68**, 143–7.
68. Maletnlema, T. N. and Bavu, J. L. (1974). Nutrition studies in pregnancy. Part I: Energy, protein and iron intake of pregnant women in Kisarawe, Tanzania. *East Africa Med. J.* **51**, 515–28.
69. Marr, J. W. (1961). A technique of carrying out individual weighed diet surveys. *Proc. Nutr. Soc.* **20**, xxxix.
70. Marr, J. W. (1965). Individual weighed dietary surveys. *Nutrition* **19**, 18–24.
71. Marr, J. W. (1971). Individual dietary surveys: purposes and methods. *Wld Rev. Nutr. Dietet.* **13**, 106–64.
72. Marr, J. W. (1981). Individual variation in dietary intake. In: *Preventive nutrition and society.* (Turner, M., ed.). Academic Press, London.
73. McFie, J. (1967). Nutrient intakes of urban dwellers in Lagos, Nigeria. *Br. J. Nutr.* **21**, 257–68.
74. Marshall, J. R., Priore, R., Graham, S., and Brasure, J. (1981). On the distation of risk estimates in multiple exposure level case-control studies. *Am. J. Epidemiol* **113**, 464–73.
75. Mertz, W. and Kelsay, J. L. (1984). Rationale and design of the Beltsville one-year dietary intake study. *Am. J. Clin. Nutr.* **40**, 1323–6.
76. Morris, J. N., Marr, J. W., and Clayton, D. G. (1977). Diet and heart: a postscript. *Br. Med. J.* **2**, 1307–14.
77. Nelson, M. and Nettleton, P. A. (1980). Dietary survey methods. 1. A semi-weighed technique for measuring dietary intake within families. *J. Hum. Nutr.* **34**, 325–48.
78. Nelson, M., Morris, J. A., Black, A. E., and Cole, T. J. (1987). Between- and within-subject variation in nutrient intake from infancy to old age. (In preparation.)
79. Nettleton, P. A., Day, K. C., and Nelson, M. (1980). Dietary survey methods. 2. A comparison of nutrient intakes within families assessed by household measures and the semi-weighed method. *J. Hum. Nutr.* **34**, 349–54.
80. Nomura, A., Hankin, J. H., and Rhoads, G. G. (1976). The reproducibility of dietary intake data in a prospective study of gastrointestinal cancer. *Am. J. Clin. Nutr.* **29**, 1432–6.
81. Norgan, N. G., Ferro-Luzzi, A., and Durnin, J. V. G. A. (1974). The energy and nutrient intake and the energy expenditure of 204 New Guinean adults. *Phil. Trans. R. Soc. Lond. B.* **268**, 309–48.
82. Nutrition Canada National Survey (1973). A report Nutrition Canada to the Department of National Health and Welfare. Information Canada, Ottawa.
83. Paul, A. A. and Southgate, D. A. T. (1978). In: *The composition of foods* (ed. R. A. McCance and E. M. Widdowson) (4th edn). HMSO, London.
84. Pekkarinen, M. (1970). Methodology in the collection of food consumption data. *Wld Rev. Nutr. Dietet.* **12**, 145–71.
85. Pietinen, P. (1985). An overview of the dietary methods used in epidemio-

logic studies on nutrition and cancer. In: *Diet and human carcinogenesis.* (Joossens, J. V., Hill, M. J., and Geboers, J. eds) pp. 235–44. Proceedings of the 3rd annual symposium of the European organization for cooperation in cancer prevention studies, Aarhus, Denmark.

86. Prentice, A. M., Whitehead, R. G., Roberts, S. B., Paul, A. A., Watkinson, M., Prentice, A., and Watkinson, A. A. (1980). Dietary supplementation of Gambian nursing mothers and lactational performance. *Lancet* ii, 886–8.
87. Prentice, A. M., Coward, W. A., Davies, H. L., *et al.* (1985). Unexpectedly low levels of energy expenditure in healthy women. *Lancet* ii, 1419–22.
88. Prentice, A. M., Black, A. E., Coward, W. A., *et al.* (1986). High levels of energy expenditure in obese women. *Br. Med. J.* **292**, 983–7.
89. Prentice, A. M. and Coward, W. A. (1986). Measurement of energy expenditure in free-living subjects using stable isotopes. *Proc. Assoc. Phys.* (in press).
90. Räsänen, L. (1982). Validity and reliability of recall methods. In: *The diet factor in epidemiological research.* (Hautvast, J. G. A. J. and Klaver, W., eds). EURO-NUT report 1, Wageningen.
91. Räsänen, L. and Pietinen, P. (1982). A short questionnaire method for evaluation of diets. *Prev. Med.* **11**, 669–76.
92. Räsänen, L., Ahola, M., Kara, R., and Uhari, M. (1985). Atherosclerosis precursors in Finnish children and adolescents. VIII Food consumption and nutrient intakes. *Acta Paediat. Scand. Suppl.* **318**, 135–53.
93. Rohan, T. E. and Potter, J. D. (1984). Retrospective assessment of dietary intake. *Am. J. Epidemiol.* **120**, 876–87.
94. Rutishauser, I. H. E. (1973). Food intake studies in pre-school children in developing countries: problems of measurement and evaluation. *Nutr. Lond.* **27**, 253–61.
95. Schofield, W. N., Schofield, C., and James, W. P. T. (1985). Basal metabolic rate. *Hum. Nutr. Clin. Nutr.* **39C** (suppl. 1), 1–96.
96. Sempos, C., Johnson, N. E., Smith, E. L., and Gilligan, C. (1985). Effects of intraindividuals and interindividual variation in repeated dietary records. *Am. J. Epidemiol.* **121**, 120–30.
97. Singh, J., Coward, W. A., Prentice, A. M., Ashford, J., Sawyer, M., Diaz, E., and Whitehead, R. G. (1988). Doubly labelled water measurements of energy expenditure in Gambian women during the agricultural season. *Proc. Nutr. Soc.* (in press).
98. Staveren, W. A. van (1974). De voedingsanamnese. In: *Informatorium voor voeding en diëtetiek.* (Hart, A. E. H., Post, G. B., and Swager, J. W., eds). Tjeenk willink, Groningen.
99. Staveren, W. A. van and Burema, J. (1985). Food consumption surveys: frustrations and expectations. *Näringsforsk.* **29**, 38–42.
100. Staveren, W. A. van, Deurenberg, P., Burema, J., and Hautvast, J. G. A. J. (1985). Validity of the 24-hour recall method repeated monthly 14 times for the assessment of the usual energy and protein intake of young adult Dutch women. In: *Food intake measurements: their validity and reproducibility.* PhD thesis, Wageningen.
101. Staveren, W. A. van, Deurenberg, P., Katan, M. B., Burema, J., Groot, L. C. P. G. M. de, and Hoffmans, M. D. A. F. (1986). Validity of the fatty acid

composition of subcutaneous fat tissue microbiopsies as an estimate of the long-term average fatty acid composition of the diet of separate individuals. *Am. J. Epidemiol.* **123**, 455–63.

102. Staveren, W. A. van, West, G. E., Hoffmans, M. D. A. F., *et al.* (1986). Comparison of contemporary and retrospective estimates of food consumption made by a dietary history method. *Am. J. Epidemiol.* **123**, 884–93.

103. Staveren, W. A. van, Deurenberg, P., Burema, J., Groot, L. C. P. G. M. de, and Hautvast, J. G. A. J. (1986). Seasonal variation in food intake, pattern of physical activity and change in body weight. *Int. J. Obesity* **10**, 133–48.

104. Steen, B., Isaksson, B., and Svanborg, A. (1977). Intake of energy and nutrients and meal habits in 70 year old males and females in Gothenburg, Sweden: a population study. *Acta Med. Scand. Suppl.* **611**, 39–86.

105. Stafanik, P. and Trulson, M. F. (1962). Determining the frequency intakes of foods in large group studies. *Am. J. Clin. Nutr.* **11**, 335–43.

106. Thompson, M., Logan, R. L., Sharman, M., Lockerbie, L., Riemersma, R. A., and Oliver, M. F. (1982). Dietary survey in 40 year old Edinburgh men. *Hum. Nutr. Appl. Nutr.* **36A**, 272–81.

107. Todd, K. S., Hudes, M., and Calloway, D. H. (1983). Food intake measurement: problems and approaches. *Am. J. Clin. Nutr.* **37**, 139–46.

108. Trulson, M. F. and McCann, M. B. (1959). Comparison of dietary survey methods. *J. Am. Diet Assoc.* **35**, 672–81.

109. Tuazon Ma, A. G. (1987). *Maternal energy requirements during pregnancy of rural Philippine women*. PhD thesis. Agricultural University, Wageningen.

110. Vet, H. C. W. de and Leeuwen, F. E. van (1986). Letter: On the reliability of historical dietary information. *Am. J. Epidemiol.* **123**, 555.

111. Wahrendorf, J. (1985). Questionnaire derived historic dietary information. In: *Diet and human carcinogenesis.* (Joossens, J. V. *et al.*, eds). Elsevier Science Publishers.

112. Walker, M. A. and Blettner, M. (1985). Comparing imperfect measures of exposure. *Am. J. Epidemiol.* **121**, 783–90.

113. Warnold, I., Carlgren, G., and Krotkiewski, M. (1978). Energy expenditure and body composition during weight reduction in hyperplastic obese women. *Am. J. Clin. Nutr.* **31**, 750–63.

114. Widdowson, E. M. (1936). A study of English diets by the individual method. Part I. Men. *J. Hyg.* **36**, 269–92.

115. Widdowson, E. M., and McCance, R. A. (1936). A study of English diets by the individual method. Part II Women. *J. Hyg.* **36**, 293–309.

116. Widdowson, E. M. (1947). A study of individual children's diets. *MRC Spec. Rep. Ser. 257.* HMSO, London.

117. Wiehl, D. G. (1942). Diets of a group of aircraft workers in Southern California. *Milbank Memorial Fund Quart.* **20**, 329–56.

118. Wiehl, D. G. and Reed, R. (1960). Development of new or improved dietary methods for epidemiological investigations. *Am. J. Publ. Hlth* **50**, 824–8.

119. Wiles, S. J., Nettleton, P. A., Black, A. E., and Paul, A. A. (1980). The nutrient content of some cooked dishes eaten in Britain: a supplementary food composition table. *J. Hum. Nutr.* **34**, 189–223.

120. Willett, W. C., Sampson, L., Stampfer, M. J. *et al.* (1985). Reproducibility

and validity of a semiquantitative food frequency questionnaire. *Am. J. Epidemiol.* **122**, 51–65.

121. World Health Organization (1985). Energy and protein requirements. *Tech. Rep. Ser.* **724**, WHO, Geneva.
122. Youland, D. M. and Eagle, A. (1976). Practices and problems in HANES, dietary data methodology. *J. Am. Diet. Assoc.* **68**, 22–5.
123. Young, C. M., Chalmers, F. W., Churchu, H. N., Clayton, M. M., Murphy, G. C., and Ticker, R. E. (1953). Subjects' estimation of food intake and calculated nutritive value of the diet. *J. Am. Diet Assoc.* **29**, 1216–20.
124. Young, C. M., Franklin, R. E., Foster, W. D., and Steele, B. F. (1953). Weekly variation in nutrient intake of young adults. *J. Am. Diet Assoc.* **29**, 459–64.
125. Young, C. M. (1959). The interview itself. *J. Am. Diet. Assoc.* **35**, 677–81.
126. Paul, A. A., Southgate, D. A. T., Currie, J. C., Jamieson, M. M., Llewelyn, B. M., Powell, J., Rothbotham, A. P. and Waterworth, M. (1977). A study of the composition of retail meat: disection into lean, separable fat and inedible portions. *J. Hum. Nutr.* **31**, 259–72.
127. US Department of Agriculture (1975). Composition of foods, *Agriculture handbook 8*, Washington, DC.
128. US Department of Agriculture (1975). Food yields summarised by different stages of preparation. *Agriculture handbook 102*. Washington, DC.

7

Technical aspects of data collection

JEAN HENDERSON SABRY AND
ELIZABETH CAMPBELL ASSELBERGS

Introduction

The technical aspects of data collection are concerned with the equipment and techniques used to measure, collect, and record food consumption.

The tools and techniques used in any survey are determined, to a large extent, by the method chosen for assessing food consumption, the population being surveyed, and the resources available. For example, weighed food records require direct measurement by a member of the survey team, the participant, or another household member; precision scales are a prerequisite. In less precise surveys, volumetric measures or recalls of estimated amounts of foods can be used. Food or portion-size models, pictures, food lists, and descriptions of standard retail products can be used to increase the accuracy and completeness of food intake reports. Reports and records may be written or dictated on tape. Methods involving written records require a certain level of literacy. Dietary history and dietary recall methods necessitate interviews, usually face-to-face, but possibly by telephone or pre-programmed computer. All information needs to be recorded, usually on forms, so that manual tabulation or computer entry and analysis are made easier.

This chapter presents the main features of the various techniques presently in use for the measurement of food consumption. Since there is no truly accurate measure of food consumption, investigators need to select those techniques and tools that satisfy the demands for precision, place least burden on interviewers' time and skills, and on the subjects' co-operation, and produce results within the time frame set. (Chapters 13 and 14.)

7.1. Advantages and disadvantages of measuring by the use of:

7.1.1. Weighing scales

If households or individuals are to weigh and record their own food consumption, each household must be provided with a good quality weighing scale for the duration of the study. If weighing is undertaken by the survey team, the number of scales required will be dictated by the number of survey teams. Scales should be sturdy enough to withstand possible careless use and frequent transport. While cost will be important, it is generally more economical to purchase good quality scales at the outset than to replace inaccurate or broken ones frequently during a survey. It is wise to have spare scales available at all times. Scales that are frequently moved should be light in weight, small in overall dimension, and fitted with a carrying case.

Capacity and sensitivity

For surveys of individual food consumption, scales with a capacity of up to 1.5 kg and a sensitivity of ± 5 g are usually adequate. Weights can then be read to the nearest 5 g. If there is specific interest in spices or condiments, which are consumed in small amounts, more sensitive scales will be necessary. For household level surveys, scales with a capacity of 5 to 10 kg and a sensitivity of ± 10 g will be required as well.

Accuracy

The accuracy of the scale at intervals over the weighing range should be checked frequently with known weights. Damaged and inaccurate scales should be repaired or replaced immediately.

Tare

Scales should include a feature that allows 'zeroing-out' of the tare weight of a food container. Newer models that allow the zeroing-out of a series of foods weighed on the same plate can markedly reduce the time required for weighing foods. However, mistakes can be made and the tare must be used with care (6.1.2).

Spring and balance scales

These are the common types of dietary scales. Generally they are not expensive. They are available from companies selling laboratory equipment. Scales with circular dials or counter weights require particular attention so that the weights of foods are properly read by directly facing the front of the dial. Spring and balance scales should have a locking device to prevent damage to the weighing mechanism during frequent transport.

Electronic digital scales

Modern electronic scales have several advantages over spring and balance scales. They are precise, the digital readout reduces error in reading weights, and they often have an automatic feature for 'zeroing-out' the weight of food containers or previously weighed foods. They are expensive, however, and require a power source or batteries. Provision must be made to have replacement batteries readily available. Maintenance of electronic scales in tropical climates may be a problem due to heat, humidity, and dust. In these situations spring or balance scales are more practical.

Electronic scales with audio-cassettes (PETRA, Cherlyn Electronics Ltd)

These newer scales might be used. The weight of the food is recorded simultaneously with descriptive data on a standard audio-cassette. Subjects do not make written records when using these scales. However, they also need re-chargeable batteries. An illustration of these scales is shown in Fig. 7.1. Figure 7.2 shows the master console being operated to use the data recorded on the cassette.

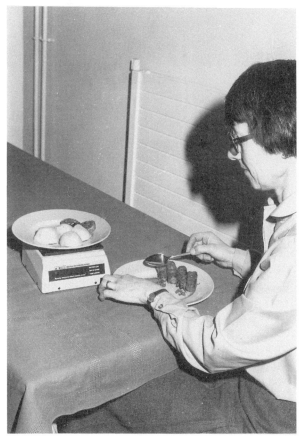

Fig. 7.1. A subject weighing and recording her food intake verbally, using the PETRA scales in Cambridge, UK.

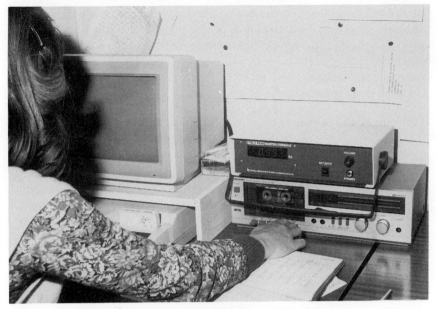

Fig. 7.2. Operating the master console for the PETRA method.

7.1.2. Volumetric containers

If the survey does not require precise weighed records of food, standardized or calibrated measurements of food may be sufficient. These measurements can be converted to weights during data processing, using volume-to-gram factors for each type of food. (6.2 and Table 6.8.)

Standardized measures

If standardized volume measures are used, they should be those most common in the area being surveyed. The metric (litre) and imperial (pint) systems are widely used. Measuring containers should be transparent and have clearly visible markings for fractions of their volumes. While the 8 oz (or 250 ml.) measuring cup is considered a standard volume in some countries, glasses are a common unit of measure in others. Standardized teaspoons and tablespoons are used as household measures in food preparation in a number of countries. Not all households will own a variety of standardized measures. Survey teams should be equipped with a set of lightweight, unbreakable, washable, standardized measures that are easy to carry.

Non-standardized measures

These refer to the variety of local measures, containers, or household spoons which may be the householder's familiar unit of measurement.

Survey teams need to be prepared to use them. Local measures may vary considerably, even between neighbouring villages, and fieldworkers will need to determine the actual volume of the local containers. Field-workers can encourage survey subjects to keep the number of non-standardized measures in use to a minimum during the survey. Caution is advised, however, since interference in the usual practice of preparing meals or serving out food could change the quantities normally used.

7.1.3. Food models, replicas, portion-size models, two-dimensional models

Food replicas, portion size models, pictures, and drawings of foods have been used to help individuals to quantify the amounts of foods eaten. In a survey, they use these as a point of reference to estimate the actual amounts eaten as fractions or multiples of the size of the model. Most studies indicate that models improve the validity of reported intake, but there is little conclusive evidence of the greater benefit of any one type. Some are thought to cause over-estimation of the consumption of certain foods while others lead to under-estimation. The size of the model may also bias results, particularly if the food portion consumed is larger or smaller than the model.[4] Estimates, aided by lifelike food models or pictures, may be made more quickly than those aided by abstract representations of amounts.[5]

Food replicas

These are three-dimensional models representing specific foods. They are life-like in size and colour and often made of plastic. Sets are commercially available in some countries, but any one set of models may not be equally appropriate in all places. The number of foods that can be represented is limited. Models of foods, culturally common in one community, may not be an appropriate selection to use elsewhere. Because the models represent actual foods, they can introduce two types of problems by: (i) suggesting that the food represented by the model was eaten; and (ii) confusing individuals who must express consumption of one food in terms of a model of another food (for example, estimating the quantity of beans in relation to a model of mashed potato).

Portion-size models

These models represent sizes of portions rather than specific foods. Thus, they avoid some of the problems already referred to in relation to food replicas. A set of such models can be made of mounds, cubes, balls, wedges, circles, and squares, used with some indicator of thickness and a selection of glasses, cups, bowls, and spoons of locally appropriate sizes. Using a graduation of sizes of each shape, rather than only one size, is less likely to bias a subject's reported consumption. It is not known whether the portion-size models are available commercially, but they can be fashioned inexpensively from wood, styrofoam, papier mâché, metal, and plastic. Local production allows the preparation of models reflecting the shapes and sizes of local foods.[6] The actual volume represented by each model should be entered into the computer so that during the survey only the code for the model needs to be recorded. Examples of portion-size models are shown in Fig. 7.3.

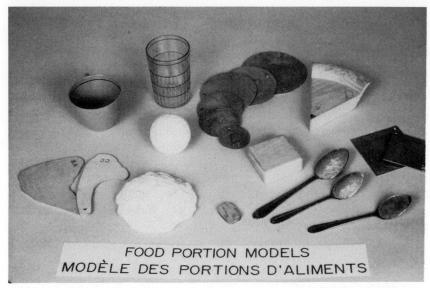

FOOD PORTION MODELS
MODÈLE DES PORTIONS D'ALIMENTS

Fig. 7.3. Portion-size food models. (Courtesy, Health and Welfare, Canada.)

Two-dimensional models

Pictures, drawings, or photographs of a wide variety of individual foods can be used by survey subjects to describe the quantities of foods eaten. All figures should be of the same scale, preferably life-size. Representation of different portion sizes of a food can help an individual to estimate the amount eaten.[3] Sets of life-sized food pictures are available commercially. However, any one set is likely to reflect the food preferences of one particular culture. The use of locally prepared drawings or photographs has obvious advantages. An example of photographic representation of three serving sizes of one food is shown in Fig. 7.4.

Three-dimensional, life-size drawings of the abstract shapes of servings of food, rather than of specific foods, also have been used with success.[5] The ease of carrying even a large set of pictures or drawings has obvious advantages over the three-dimensional types of food models already mentioned.

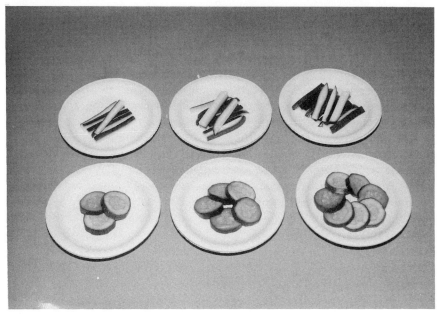

Fig. 7.4. Photographic representation of three serving sizes of zucchini (courgette) shown for two forms of the vegetable. (Courtesy of J. H. Hankin, University of Hawaii.)

7.1.4. Average portion sizes

Surveys concerned with the overall quality of diets or the frequency of consumption of certain foods often ask subjects to report only the number of average servings of a food consumed. The size of average servings may need to be defined by weight, volume, or photograph so that both the interviewer and the subject use the same amount as a reference. Data on average portions of food consumed by persons in different age/sex categories are sometimes available from data collected in other surveys.[7,9] Typical serving sizes are often given in food composition tables.

Food counts

Foods such as fruits, eggs, candy bars, and pre-portioned servings of foods, for example, bread slices, cartons of yogurt, bottled carbonated beverages, or beer and packages of frozen meals, often can be reported as units or counts (Table 6.8). Larger than average fruits can be reported as multiples of average ones, although it is difficult for most people to express the relative size of one fruit or vegetable in relation to another. For foods of a standard size, counts may be the most accurate unit of reporting. Where current local market prices are known, consumption of a food can be reported by its cost and then converted to a weight.

7.1.5. Food photography

For prospective studies of food consumption there are promising new approaches using food photography. In one procedure, photographs of meals consumed by the survey subject are projected alongside standard slides showing a variety of portion sizes of the same foods.[2] The other procedure uses a computer to convert photographs of foods into volumetric and weight equivalents.[10] Food photography avoids the use of scales or other measures and reduces the disruption resulting from weighed and measured surveys. However, the cost of cameras and films will probably prevent their use in any but small scale precision studies, in the near future.

7.2. Advantages and disadvantages of collecting data by:

7.2.1. Observation

Direct observation and measurement

With direct observation, trained fieldworkers observe and record, by weight or volume, the food consumed by the survey subject. Usually the fieldworker is present from the subject's first food intake, in the morning, until the last one in the evening. A more limited form of observation occurs when the fieldworker is present at meal times and obtains information from the subject on foods eaten outside the home during the day. The greatest advantage of direct observation and measurement is the quality of data collected. Measurements and descriptions of foods are more likely to be accurate and consistent. Observer measurement places less burden on any subject than does self-reporting (6.3). If the survey population is illiterate or unable to measure and record food intake accurately, there is no good alternative to observed measurements. The disadvantages of observer measurement are intrusiveness and cost and their presence affects the social environment in which food is consumed. Survey subjects may change their food consumption pattern in an attempt to please or impress. Daily activities and the time available for food preparation and consumption may also be influenced. In some cultures, for example, traditional courtesies may require rural women to forgo agricultural work when there is a visitor (the fieldworker) in the household. Direct observation is costly in terms of personnel. One person cannot fully observe and record the food intake of more than one individual or household at a time unless they are living closely together. Travel and accommodation costs are also likely to be substantial (13.4).

Unobtrusive observation

In some situations food intake may be observed and measured without the individual being aware of the observation. This is possible in institutions where the type and amount of food served and the amount left uneaten can be measured in a way that does not directly involve the individual. This method has been used in clinics, hospitals, nursing homes, and with students in residence halls.

7.2.2. Respondent measurement and recording

The alternative to observer measurement of food intake is for the subjects to do it themselves (6.1, 6.2), or in the case of children, it would be done by another household member. Careful instruction in record-keeping and weighing or other measurement of food quantities is essential. If records are kept for several days, visits by fieldworkers to monitor the food records and sustain the subject's interest may be necessary. Recording by the subject places considerable demand on their time, especially if the food intake must be weighed.

Written and dictated records

Records may be kept by writing or by dictating to a recording device such as a cassette tape recorder. Written records are more common. They are less expensive, but subjects must be literate and physically able to write. Taped records are costly due to the initial cost of the tape recorder and the time required to transcribe the tapes. It has been observed that dictated records tend to be completed during the meal and written records to be made later in the day.[1] Taped records may be less disruptive to the subjects' daily routine than written records and especially useful if subjects are unable to write.

7.2.3. Interviews

Interviewing is used in retrospective methods of obtaining dietary intake information such as the dietary history, daily recall, and food frequency (6.5). Interviews make few demands on the subject other than the time required for the interview and their effort of recalling food intake. The food consumption environment at home is not altered. It is important for interviewers to be well-informed about the foods available in the survey community, their cooking and food preparation methods, and the food habits and customs.

The manner and skills of the interviewer are important for the success of an interview. Respondents are more likely to feel at ease if the interviewer has a friendly and courteous manner, observes local forms of greeting and personal address, and is dressed inconspicuously in a way that does not offend local customs.

The interview should begin with a brief introduction and proceed in a straightforward fashion. The interviewer should stress the need for reporting the food intake as accurately as possible. It is important to allow subjects sufficient time to consider their answers. If pressed to answer a question too quickly they may react by inventing answers or saying they cannot remember. The interviewer should keep irrelevant conversation to a minimum and keep the interview to the reporting of food intake information or answers for other questions on the interview form. Interviewers must be extremely careful to ask neutral questions to prevent any bias in the answers. They should not show approval or disapproval of any replies made. They must avoid asking questions which suggest the answers.

The structure of the interview will depend on whether the procedure is the dietary history (6.7), the daily food recall (6.6), or food frequencies (6.8). Careful training and monitoring of interviewers is necessary to minimize differences in style and to ensure that they follow the given protocol.

Interviews in the home

There are certain advantages to conducting dietary interviews in the subjects' homes. It is convenient and may encourage participation in the survey. The familiar environment may improve the recall of food consumed. Food items, food packages with labels, and the usual household measures can be shown to the interviewer. A disadvantage to interviewing at home is the opportunity for interruptions from children, visitors, or telephone calls. In small homes it may not be possible for the fieldworker to interview the survey subject alone and the presence of other persons in the room may distract or influence the answers given. With home interviews, a considerable amount of interviewer time may be spent in travel between homes and in repeated visits to find the subjects at home.

Interviews at clinics

In population surveys, the survey team may set up a temporary clinic in each locality. In studies conducted by personnel at health centres or universities, subjects often come to a clinic for interview. In the clinic they are free from outside distractions, but may feel somewhat ill-at-ease in a strange environment. If the survey provides transport for the subjects to the clinic centre, survey travel costs may be similar to those for home interviews. Nevertheless clinic interviews are more convenient for the survey team. Survey materials including food models and reporting forms are at hand. Interviewer time is not spent in travel. Supervision and monitoring of interviewer performance can be carried out more readily in a clinic than at a home interview.

Telephone interviews

Telephone interviews have the advantage of relatively low cost since neither survey respondents or interviewers travel to an interview site. The survey sample can be selected without regard to the convenience of location. However, samples selected by telephone may not be representative of the population since less privileged groups are less likely than others to have telephones. In telephone interviews, it is difficult for respondents to convey information on food items and quantities. This difficulty may be overcome by providing respondents before the interview with two-dimensional food portion models.[8] Telephone interviews cannot be as prolonged as direct interviews. Telephone interviews are particularly suitable for food frequency surveys and for surveys to obtain information about the consumption of specific food items (6.6.3).

In computer-assisted telephone interviews, the telephone interviewer enters the respondent's reply directly into a computer terminal. This saves time by combining the interview with data entry and can reduce errors by eliminating one step in data processing. Computer assisted telephone interviews are feasible if the interview is brief and the collected information is fairly simple.

Little is known about the difference in dietary information collected by telephone interview compared with that collected in a personal interview. There is some indication from surveys for other purposes that in telephone interviews there is less tendency for persons to give socially desirable responses than is the case in face-to-face interview.[11] However, in depth probing is more difficult to accomplish in the telephone interview. Although the interviewer's personal characteristics are less likely to bias a telephone interview, the interviewer must still be careful to avoid conveying, by comment or tone of voice, approval or disapproval of the respondent's reply.

Computer interview

Dietary information may be collected directly by computer, using specially designed programs. One such program has been used with clinic patients.[12] The questions asked must be neutral and the choices for replies must be clearly presented. Computer interviewing avoids the cost of interview personnel, but adds the cost of computer hardware and software. In other fields of study it has been found that many persons react favourably to computer interviewing, although a small number have difficulty in using the computer. Answers to sensitive questions may be more honest than with face-to-face interviews.

7.3. Ethical considerations

Investigators have an obligation to be ethically responsible in all dealings with survey participants. Subjects should be fully informed about the nature of the project and what their participation will involve before they consent to participate. Consent should be given freely, without coercion or inducement, and they should be informed that they are allowed to withdraw from the study and to withhold information about themselves.

Personal information, such as that collected in food consumption surveys, should be treated with strict confidentiality. Code numbers, rather than names, should be used for identification, unless there is an explicit plan to provide feedback to the participants. Many countries have legal requirements for the storage and retrieval of personal information obtained from volunteers. These should be taken into account when planning the survey or research study.

All studies or surveys with human subjects should have the approval of the ethical committee of the institution or agency involved in the survey.

Many jurisdictions require a research licence or survey permit. Investigators are responsible for finding out whether or not a research licence is necessary and for obtaining it from the appropriate authority.

References

1. Arab, L., Schlierf, G., Schellenberg, B., and Kohlmeier, M. (1979). A cost–benefit assessment approach to nutritional protocol selection. *Prohl. Ernähr. Lebensm. Wiss.* **6**, 131–44.
2. Elwood, P. C. and Bird, G. (1983). A photographic method of diet evaluation. *Human Nutr.* **37A**, 474–7.
3. Hankin, J. H. (1986). A diet history method for research, clinical and community use. *J. Am. Diet Assoc.* **86**, 868–72.
4. Karlström, A. B., Abrahamsson, L., Hadell, K., Skoog, E., Barkeling, B., and Wirfalt, E. (1985). Användning av livsmedelsmodeller i kostintervjuer. Näringsforsk. **29**, 52–9.
5. Kircaldy-Hargreaves, L., Lynch, G. W., and Santor, C. (1980). Assessment of the validity of four food models. *J. Can. Diet Assoc.* **41**, 102–11.
6. Moore, M. C., Judlin, B. C., and Kennemur, P. M. (1967). Using graduated food models in taking dietary histories. *J. Am. Diet Assoc.* **51**, 447–50.
7. Pao, E. M., Fleming, K. H., Guenther, P. M., and Mickle, S. J. (1982). Foods commonly eaten by individuals: Amount per day and per eating occasion. Washington: Consumer Nutrition Center, Human Nutrition Information

Service, United States Department of Agriculture. Home Economics Research Report No 44.

8. Posner, B. M., Borman, C. L., Morgan, J. L., Borden, W. S., and Ohls, J. C. (1982). The validity of a telephone-administered 24-hour dietary recall methodology. *Am. J. Clin. Nutr.* **36**, 546–53.
9. Sabry, J. H. and Cherry, A. (1985). Portion size of some commonly consumed foods. *J. Can. Diet Assoc.* **46**, 59–63.
10. Sevenhuysen, G. (1985). Image processing to measure individual food consumption. 13th International Congress of Nutrition, Brighton.
11. Tyebjee, T. T. (1979). Telephone survey methods: The state of the art. *J. Marketing* **43**, 68–78.
12. Witschi, J. (1982). Interviewing by computer. In: Beal, V. A., Laus, M. J., eds. Proceedings of the symposium on dietary collection, analysis and significance. *Res. Bull. No. 675*, pp. 12–14. Massachusetts Agricultural Experiment Station, Amherst.

8

Conversion into nutrients

ALISON A. PAUL AND DAVID A. T. SOUTHGATE
(WITH CONTRIBUTIONS FROM TIM COLE
AND KEN DAY)

Introduction

Most, but by no means all, measurements of food consumption are undertaken so that the nutrient intake of individuals or groups can be calculated. As has been stated in Chapter 6 the second important component of the study is knowledge of the nutrient composition of the foods that have been consumed. In most studies, particularly of free-living individuals and with large numbers of subjects, one or more of the published food composition tables will be used (8.2). However in many other instances the information required is not available in food tables, and direct analysis of foods or diets becomes a necessity.

8.1. Direct analysis

8.1.1. The need for direct analysis

It is unlikely that the investigators will be needing, or have the facilities, to construct a food composition table for a wide range of nutrients entirely from scratch. A more typical need for new food analysis would be where values are required for a constituent not given in existing tables. Examples are: certain trace elements, food additives, and contaminants; a nutrient where information is lacking for a number of foods, such as for fatty acids; where improved methods of analysis and understanding of biological availability lead to existing values being outdated, (e.g. dietary fibre and folic acid).

In other instances there may be no existing information on the foods actually consumed, particularly for cooked foods. A food table appropriate for that particular study would have to be prepared (8.6). For metabolic studies food tables are not sufficiently accurate and direct analyses of the nutrients of interest are necessary.

In multi-centre studies a comparable analysis of the constituents in the major foods in each of the centres may be considered necessary, even if only as a check on the comparability of the different food composition tables being used. Because a detailed discussion of the many aspects of food sampling and analysis is outside the scope of this manual, the reader is referred to Greenfield and Southgate[12] and Southgate.[22]

Food analysis is costly and time consuming, therefore a sensible balance should be drawn between making use of existing values and starting new analyses. Critical scrutiny of literature values is necessary before they are adopted, and the requirements will vary depending on whether, for example, energy and major constituents of foods are the purpose of the study, or whether it is a detailed investigation into a particular constituent about which little is known. The intake of some nutrients (vitamin C, sodium, folates) cannot be estimated with acceptable accuracy by calculation from food tables and if these nutrients are crucial to the study, direct analysis of replicate diets would be essential.

Requirements for the production of good quality food composition data are summarized in Table 8.1.

Table 8.1. Details ideally required for good quality food composition data: description and analysis of samples

General heading	Details required
Name of food	Common name, with local synonyms.
	Scientific taxonomic names with variety where known.
Origin of food	Plant foods: locality where grown, with details of soil conditions and fertilizer treatments.
	Animal products: locality and method of husbandry and slaughter (where applicable).
Nature of sample collected	Place and time of collection. Number of samples collected; whether purchased retail.
	State in which it was purchased, e.g., raw, prepared, deep frozen, pre-packed, etc.
Treatment of samples before analysis	Conditions and length of storage.
	Preparative treatment, including details of material discarded as waste.
	Method of cooking (where applicable).
Analysis	Details of material analysed.
	Analytical methods used, with appropriate references and details of any modifications used.
Method of expression of results*	Statistical treatment of analytical values.
	Whether expressed on the basis of 'as purchased', 'edible matter' or 'dry matter'.

*Whenever results are expressed on a basis other than fresh weight, details should be given so that the results can be calculated back to this basis.

8.1.2. Food samples

These should be both representative of those available or to be consumed by the population concerned. The portion analysed should also be representative of the particular food in question. Ideally a number of samples of each item, at least ten, should be analysed, but frequently a compromise has to be made, and a single composite made up of ten samples is analysed. There should be a protocol which includes such details as the number and size of samples, their distribution between different outlets or numbers of subjects and full post-collection handling procedures. Where background knowledge is available, account should be taken of factors such as variety, seasonality, or area where grown. In addition the food should be obtained in the form in which it is usually consumed and thus relate directly to the stage at which it is being measured in the dietary study.

8.1.3. Presentation in the laboratory

Data quality will depend to a considerable extent on the way the food is handled before and on arrival in the laboratory. Foods are subject to attack by microorganisms or internal agents such as enzymes. They may undergo chemical alteration due to the action of heat, light, oxygen, moisture, and contaminants such as metal instruments and catalysts. Prior to analysis they need to be homogenized and blended, a process which renders nutrients labile through exposure to destructive agents.

8.1.4. The analysis

The most appropriate analytical procedures must be selected to reflect most closely the nutritonal value of the food for man. For many nutrients, a number of procedures are available which give comparable results. Procedures developed most recently require the use of extensive instrumentation and therefore of capital investment. Other procedures often give similar results, but have been discontinued because of their time consuming nature. Methods suitable for use have been summarized, with bibliographical details, by Southgate.[22]

8.2. Use of food composition tables—general considerations

8.2.1. Food composition tables for different parts of the world

In the great majority of cases, food consumption data will be converted into energy and nutrients by using food composition tables. Tables are now available for most major areas of the world, ranging in scope from those covering continents, to specific tables for an area within a single country. Table 8.2 summarizes some of the main tables, numerous others are listed in the recent INFOODS, *International directory of food composition*[13] and fuller details are given in the earlier *FAO annotated bibliography.*[8] Further information on European tables is provided by West.[26] As well as in the printed books, several tables are now available in computer readable form.

8.2.2. Comparisons between tables

Variability in food composition

For any given food appearing in more than one of these tables, there will invariably be differences in the constituents presented. These serve to highlight one of the most important facts of food composition tables. Foods do vary in composition, and people who regard the values as immutable constants are deceiving themselves. Differences are usually due to the natural biological variation in the composition of any food, as usually it is possible to analyse relatively few samples. Entries are sometimes based on just one sample of a food. Consequently the low reliance of such values should be given attention. Raw basic foods have considerable variability, but once local cooking procedures are added into the food tables, even wider differences can be expected. Manufactured foods may also show marked variability, particularly with regard to added minerals and vitamins. For these reasons, it is essential for any table to document its sources of information, so that the users can decide for themselves on the reliability of values given. It is common for the same information to be presented in many different tables, by being taken from an earlier or more comprehensive publication. Provided the source is given, this is acceptable in many cases, but unless carefully scrutinized, incorrect or outdated values can be perpetuated beyond their useful life.

Modes of expression

It is also important to remember that food tables prepared by different authorities may adopt different principles in a number of important aspects, and older tables still in use may contain conventions that have been superseded. The introductory text and explanatory notes should always be read before using the tables. Here language presents a greater problem, than the tables themselves. To overcome this a start has been made by translating the introductions and comparing modes of expression in many European tables.[2, 3]

A discussion of the most notable of the pitfalls in using tables of food composition now follows.

1. Energy value, carbohydrates, and fibre: virtually all tables present

Table 8.2. Summary of the main food composition tables covering different parts of the world. (Adapted from INFOODS.[13])

Continent	Area tables	Individual country's tables and year of publication*
Africa	Food composition tables for use in Africa (Wu Leung et al, 1968).	Cameroon (1966), Egypt (1985), Ethiopia (1968), Ghana (1969), Congo (1968), Senegal (1961), South Africa (1982), Zambia (1971).
Asia	Food composition table for use in East Asia (Wu Leung et al, 1972).	Burma (1967), China (1982), India (1971), Indonesia (1981), Japan (1982), Korea (1981), Malaysia (1982), Pakistan (1985), Philippines (1980), Sri Lanka (1979), Thailand (1981).
Europe	See Eurofoods directory (West, 1985).	Tables from 22 countries.
Middle East	Food composition tables for the Near East (FAO and USDA, 1982).	Arabian Gulf States (1985), Israel (1982), Turkey (1966).
North America	Composition of foods — raw, processed, prepared (USDA, 1976–86).	Canada (1985), Caribbean (1974), Cuba (1979), Haiti (1965), Mexico (1980).
Oceana	Tables of composition of Australian foods (Thomas and Corden, 1977).	Pacific Islands (1983).
South America	INCAP-ICNND food composition table for use in Latin America (Wu Leung and Flores, 1961).	Bolivia (1984), Brazil (1977), Chile (1979), Colombia (1978), Dominican Republic (1971), Ecuador (1965), Guatemala (1968), Peru (1975), Surinam (1968), Venezuela (1983).

*For publication details and other tables see FAO, Infoods, and West.[8,13,26,29–31]

available or metabolizable energy values, but they are likely to use different factors to calculate this from the protein, fat, carbohydrate, and alcohol contents of the foods. The principle of the treatment of the unavailable carbohydrate (or dietary fibre) fraction gives rise to the largest international differences. The McCance and Widdowson tables[17] have established the British tradition of the direct measurement of both available and unavailable carbohydrate, and they use the factors 16 kJ/g (3.75 kcal/g) for available carbohydrate expressed as monosaccharide. In contrast, tables prepared by US and FAO authorities give values only for crude fibre, and use different energy conversion factors for the carbohydrates in different foods, the carbohydrates having been obtained 'by difference' (that is 100 minus the sum of the water, protein, fat, and ash content of the food). The various approaches are summarized in Fig. 8.1.

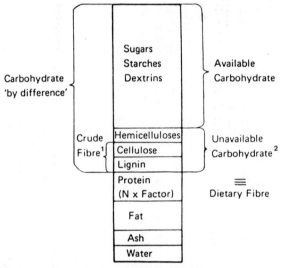

Fig. 8.1. Proximate constituents in foods showing the different ways of expressing carbohydrates.

[1] This fraction may include small amounts of hemicelluloses.
[2] As originally defined this included the non-carbohydrate lignin.

British tables now also use a single factor for all foods for protein, 17 kJ/g (4 kcal/g), and fat, 37 kJ/g (9 kcal/g), as recommended by the Royal Society.[21] Tables of US origin have retained the Atwater system[15] of specific energy factors for different types of foods. In practice, the use of the various principles gives different calculated energy contents for some individual foods (see Table 8.3), but differences are small when considering the diet as a whole. Further discussion of the derivation of energy conversion factors is given by Widdowson.[27]

2. Protein: this is conventionally calculated from the total nitrogen in

Table 8.3. Comparisons of energy values of selected foods using different conversion factors

	kcal/100 g			kJ/100 g		
	Royal Society*	Atwater system†	Percentage difference	Royal Society*	Atwater system†	Percentage difference
Bread, white	233	250	+7.3	991	1047	+5.7
Rice, polished, boiled	123	121	−1.6	522	507	−2.9
Butter	740	723	−2.3	3041	3025	−0.5
Cheese, cheddar	406	407	+0.2	1682	1703	+1.2
Milk, whole	65	65	0	272	273	+0.4
Vegetable oils	899	883	−1.8	3696	3695	0
Apples, raw	46	56	+21.7	196	233	+18.9
Bananas	79	104	+31.6	337	434	+28.8
Oranges	35	48	+37.1	150	203	+35.3
Peanuts/groundnuts	570	575	+0.9	2364	2408	+1.9
Potatoes, old, boiled	80	93	+16.3	343	389	+13.4

*Protein×17 kJ/g (4 kcal/g), fat×37 kJ/g (9 kcal/g), available carbohydrate as monosaccharide×16 kJ/g (3.75 kcal/g), as used by Paul and Southgate.[17]
†Individual factors for protein, fat and total carbohydrate, calculated by difference, as given by FAO/WHO and Merrill and Watt.[10,15]

the food, and while the average nitrogen content of proteins is about 16 per cent, giving rise to a factor of 6.25, there is some variation with different food proteins ranging from 15.7 to 19.3 per cent. A few food tables use a consistent factor of 6.25 for all foods, but most of them single out individual factors of between 5.7 and 5.95 for various cereals, 5.3 for most nuts and 6.38 for milk, assigning 6.25 to the remaining foods.[10] In the 1985 report on energy and protein requirements,[11] however, such detail was considered unnecessary when viewing the overall protein intake, which is measured as nitrogen, in relation to protein needs.

3. Vitamin A and carotene: these are undoubtedly the most problematical in terms of its expression in food tables. First, there are differences with the older usage of international units being replaced by micrograms. Second, in various tables different assumptions are made about the equivalence of total carotene to β carotene, and then of β carotene to retinol equivalents. In spite of internationally accepted definitions of 1 IU vitamin A$=0.3$ μg β carotene and 1 μg retinol equivalent$=6$ μg β carotene or 12 μg of other carotenoids, not all food tables conform. In fact some tables prepared before the adoption of the definitions are still being used. This variety of expression results in descriptions such as 'vitamin A potency', 'vitamin A value', 'β carotene equivalent', 'retinol', and 'carotene'.

4. Nicotinic acid* and tryptophan: nicotinic acid is another vitamin for which 'equivalence' values are beginning to be used. Such values are essential if calculated nutrient intakes are to be correctly related to the recommended dietary amounts. For this, the contribution from tryptophan (60 mg tryptophan $\equiv$ 1 mg nicotinic acid) should be added to the nicotinic acid in the diet. In the British table,[17] to ease this calculation the tryptophan, divided by 60, is given for each food even though the evidence is insufficient to suggest that this ratio applies with equal precision to every food. Where no information is given, the tryptophan can be calculated approximately by taking 1.4 per cent of the animal protein and 1 per cent of the vegetable protein in the diet.

8.2.3. Updating of food tables

1. Available information; the range of foods available for consumption is never static. New varieties of plants become commercially important and marketing, distribution, and consumption patterns change so that food tables need regular updating. It is difficult for tables to be

*The preferred term is nicotinic acid,[14] but it is also known as niacin, nicotinamide, PP factor (pellagra preventing).

constantly revised as they are substantial publications requiring much time, effort, and expense to compile. Fortunately the majority of the information on well-known nutrients in basic foods would not be expected to change a great deal in newer editions. It is for new foods or foods that have changed that revision is often needed (8.3.3) and for those nutrients where analytical methodology is improving. Particular examples are for unavailable carbohydrates (dietary fibre) and folic acid, where new information about the digestibility and availability of various forms to the human is becoming known. Information, however, is still far from complete. Analytical procedures are also showing that values given in tables for dietary fibre and folate may be incorrect. For fatty acids, recent analyses made on many foods have not yet (in 1987) been incorporated into all tables. As great variability is shown, particularly with manufactured foods relying on mixtures of fats and oils, it is difficult to include 'typical' values in any food table. Often new analytical data on foods and nutrients are available from manufacturers before they can be included in more readily usable tables.[18]

2. Secular trends in nutrient intake: comparisons of nutrient intake over several years can be confusing because of changes in food composition data, given in updated editions of food tables. For example, many fat and iron values are lower in the fourth edition of McCance and Widdowson's tables compared with the third, while vitamin A and riboflavin values in key foods are higher. These differences are large enough to affect the calculated total nutrient intake of specific groups of people and also the average intake of the British population.[18]

3. Symbols and abbreviations: particular attention should always be given to these and especially to the dash ($-$). This one is most frequently overlooked and misused. The dash does *not* mean '0' or zero. It means that no information is available, although it is probable from the nature of the food that some of the nutrient is present. An approximate value from a related food, or even an informed guess, should be used in place of the ($-$) and the resulting calculations treated with the caution they deserve.

8.2.4. Accuracy when using food composition tables

Many factors influence accuracy when using the food tables. These influences are shown in Fig. 8.2.

The degree of accuracy of the food composition tables also influences the ultimate accuracy of calculated nutrient intakes. In general, however, the variability in measuring food intakes is greater than the variability in the food composition itself, even though both are difficult to quantify because of the numerous factors involved in both of these components.

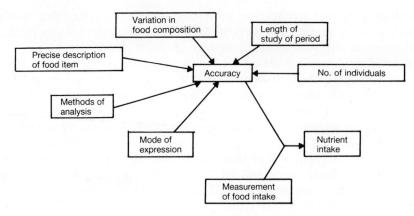

Fig. 8.2. Factors influencing the accuracy when using food tables.

8.2.5. Statistical information on variability of food composition

This is given in a few food composition tables, although it is now included in the more recent comprehensive publications.[9,25] Perhaps because of the intricacies involved, little use, so far, appears to have been made of this information in dietary calculations. The following outlines some of the general principles.

> The daily intake of a specified nutrient is the sum of the weight of food multiplied by the mean nutrient content of food, for each food eaten during the day.   (A)

> The variance of this nutrient intake is the sum of: (weight of food multiplied by the standard deviation (SD) of nutrient content of food)^2 (B)

The SD of the daily nutrient intake is the square root of this value.

The variation in nutrient content can be expressed as a coefficient of variation (CV). This is the SD divided by the daily nutrient intake (A). In the simplest case, where equal weights of, for example, the number (n) of foods are eaten during the day and if the CV for each food's nutrient composition is the same, then the CV for the daily nutrient intake is $CV/\sqrt{n}$. In practice, exactly equal weights of different foods are not eaten and each food's CV will be different.

Therefore, put in algebraic terms, if each food has a weight eaten of w_i and a food table nutrient value m_i with SD s_i, then the CV for the daily nutrient intake is given by:

$$\frac{\sqrt{(\Sigma w_i^2 s_i^2)}}{(\Sigma w_i m_i)} \qquad (C)$$

In general, this value gets smaller as n increases.

Thus the greater n is, that is the more foods that are eaten during the day, the less important the uncertainty in the food table values becomes.

Conversely in a typical African diet where the number of foods eaten is small (perhaps 3 to 5) and where individual foods vary widely in their water content, the uncertainty attached to the daily intake can be huge.

Continuing this idea, a series of daily values for an individual subject can be combined using the information on variation.

If each day's intake is d_j, with a SD of t_j (derived as the numerator of (C)), the best estimate for the subject's intake is

$$\frac{\Sigma(d_j/t_j^2)}{\Sigma(1/t_j^2)} \tag{D}$$

In this expression each daily value d_j is given a weighting inversely as the square of its SD t_j.

This same formula can be used for combining different individuals, or for a combination of days and individuals.

Confidence intervals are a useful way of expressing the uncertainty due to variability in food consumption, that is a range of values for the daily intake which has a specified chance of including the true value. A 95 per cent confidence interval ranges from the mean minus two SDs to the mean plus two SDs, while a 68 per cent confidence interval is given by the mean plus and minus one SD.

As an example, consider a confidence interval for the fat intake of an individual consuming 250 ml of milk. The mean fat content of the milk is 3.34 g/100 g and the standard deviation 0.18 g/100 g, as given in food number 01-077 in the USDA *Composition of foods*.[25]

$$\text{Mean fat intake} = 250 \times \frac{3.34}{100} = 8.35\,\text{g}$$

$$\text{SD of intake} \quad = 250 \times \frac{0.18}{100} = 0.45\,\text{g}$$

$$\begin{aligned}\text{95 per cent confidence interval} &= 8.35 \pm 2 \times 0.45\,\text{g} \\ &= 7.45 \text{ to } 9.25\,\text{g}\end{aligned}$$

The confidence interval of dietary intake from more than one food is calculated from the sum of the intakes of each component food. Continuing the above example:

The 95 per cent confidence interval for an individual's fat intake from 250 ml milk (composition as above) and 15 g butter (mean fat 81.11 g/ 100 g, SD 1.57, USDA item No. 01-001 1974) would be:

$$\text{Mean fat intake} \quad = 250 \times \frac{3.34}{100} + 15 \times \frac{81.11}{100} = 20.52 \text{ g}$$

$$(\text{SD of fat intake})^2 = \left(250 \times \frac{0.18}{100}\right)^2 + \left(15 \times \frac{1.57}{100}\right)^2 = (0.51 \text{ g})^2$$

$$\begin{aligned}\text{95 per cent confidence interval} &= 20.52 \pm 2 \times 0.51 \\ &= 19.50 \text{ to } 21.54 \text{ g fat}\end{aligned}$$

These calculations only apply on the assumption that the composition of the food shows random variation between samples. Such a situation may not, however, always occur in practice. For example in a dietary estimation of vitamin C, individual subjects may consume a particular brand of a food or drink fortified to a high level, or may always cook their vegetables in a way that either preserves the vitamin C or accelerates its destruction. In some African communities, local food mixtures will be made in characteristic ways by different individuals and foods such as gruels or steamed cereals may be characteristically cooked to different degrees of moisture content. Owing to this, the overall standard deviation of the food composition found in samples collected from the whole community will not be applicable for particular individuals.

8.2.6. Comparison of calculated and analysed diets

Guidance in this area can only be general because the number of studies where this accuracy has been tested experimentally is very limited.[17] One critical factor is how appropriate the food table is for the study in question and conclusions have been drawn discrediting food tables unnecessarily harshly because the precise items consumed were not in the tables. Where more controlled studies have been conducted, for example under metabolic balance conditions, the agreement between calculated and analysed values for protein, carbohydrate, energy, potassium, calcium, magnesium, and phosphorus is usually between 5–10 per cent. Calculated fat intakes often show greater discrepancies, but this can sometimes be attributed to the method of analysis for fat. The amount of fat included in meat eaten is a particular area causing large variations. Calculated intakes of sodium and iron may differ greatly from analysed values because of variations in added salt and contamination, respectively. Vitamin C intakes can also show big discrepancies due to natural variation in fruits and vegetables and more particularly to losses on cooking. The food table values for this vitamin may, however, represent rather ideal circumstances not always encountered in practice. There is little information about other vitamins, but vitamins A and D which show high variability in food content, can be expected to show less good agreement than many of the B vitamins. Amino acids show quite good agreement while fatty acids show considerable variation due to differences in the manufactured food items.

One can summarize with an apt quotation of Widdowson and McCance.[28] 'There are two schools of thought about food tables. One tends to regard the figures in them as having the accuracy of atomic weight determinations, the other dismisses them as valueless on the grounds that a food may be so modified by the soil, the season or its rate of growth that no figure can be a reliable guide to its composition. The truth, of course, lies somewhere between these points of view.'

8.3. Use of the tables — at a practical level

8.3.1. Coding of foods

The main use of food tables in the dietary survey will be to assign nutrient composition values to the food items used in the survey. Since a great many of the nutrient calculations are likely to be done using a computer, the first process is to identify each food item with the code number it has in composition tables. The way in which this is done is described in 9.1.2.

8.3.2. Food names

For most of the food items, provided the tables used are appropriate to the situation, the coding will be relatively straightforward. Coders must be familiar with the food descriptions given and should not use an index of non-specific names and numbers alone. Where food tables are arranged by food group, use of an alphabetical index is also necessary, as foods may be listed in a group different from the one expected. Systematic (Latin) names are particularly useful in international comparisons especially for vegetables, fruit, cereals, and fish. Local synonyms may not always be given in the tables, but can be used with appropriate preliminary knowledge.

8.3.3. Foods not listed in the tables

Inevitably, there will be foods used that are not listed in the tables and this is when the most skill and experience is required. If the food cannot be related to another one in the local table, values must either be adopted from another food composition table, taken from the literature, or requested from the food manufacturers, if appropriate. Ideally, where no suitable information exists and facilities are available, the food should be analysed, especially if it has been consumed frequently. It should *never* be left out of the dietary calculation.

8.3.4. Recipes

One of the most frequent areas of limited knowledge is in determining the value of foods cooked in different ways and by more complex and varied recipes than those given in the tables. One method is to construct one's own recipe from the ingredients given; enter these ingredients into the dietary record (for those with no cooking loss); and create, as is usually done, a new code number to add to the tables.

This exercise is made considerably easier with computer calculations.[6] However, another method[17] is as follows:

1. The weights of the raw ingredients are used to calculate the total amounts of nutrients in the recipe/food mix/meal. A correction for wastage due to ingredients left on utensils and in the vessels used in preparation is made at this stage.

2. The weight of the raw mix is then measured, using a scale with an accuracy of ± 1 g, though a less accurate scale may be used if the total weight of ingredients is over 500 g.

3. The mix is then cooked and reweighed. (A minor correction to allow for the difference between weighing it hot and at room temperature is not usually necessary.)

4. The difference in weight is accounted for by water and the composition of the cooked mix is calculated as follows:

   (a) divide the total nutrients in the mix, calculated from the raw ingredients, by the weight of the cooked mix and multiply by 100;

   (b) the water content of the raw ingredients minus the loss in weight on cooking, divided by the weight of the cooked mix gives the water content of the cooked mix, if it is required.

An example is:

Egg custard

	Amount in recipe g	Amounts contributed		
Ingredient		Protein g	Fat g	Carbohydrate, etc. g
Milk	500	16.5	19.0	23.5
Egg	100	12.3	10.9	Tr
Sugar	30	0	0	31.5
Vanilla essence	To taste	Ignored for calculation		
Total in recipe (a)	630	28.8	29.9	55.0
Cooked weight	500			
Composition of cooked custard (per 100 g) (b)	—	5.8	6.0	11.0

(a) = sum of nutrients in ingredients.
(b) = (a) divided by cooked weight $\times$ 100 ((28.8/500)$\times$100=5.8).

If some of the ingredients are left in the mixing bowl or not used then the (a) values should be multiplied by weight used divided by weight of total ingredients.

This principle can be used for any recipe or food mix where the only change on cooking is loss of water. Where fat is gained in a fried food, then the only safe method is to analyse for fat content before and after cooking; the rest of the nutrients can then be calculated. Where appropriate, vitamin losses should be taken into account using factors such as those given in the introduction to McCance and Widdowson's *The composition of foods*.[17]

8.3.5. Manufactured foods

The second major area of limited knowledge is likely to be with manufactured foods. Most manufacturers are willing to provide nutrient information and indeed, recent practices give this on labels or packets which eases the coder's task considerably. However, such data may be calculated from ingredients and be based on different concepts particularly for carbohydrate and energy (8.2.2). Recalculation of some values would be necessary to make them compatible with the remainder of the food table.

8.3.6. Creation of a supplementary food table for the dietary study

Many studies are almost certain to need values for extra items consumed by their particular group of subjects. Depending on the food code system given in the original food table, these can be either added on to the end, or slotted into appropriate food groups. It is advisable to distinguish them with a prefix or some other identity. This is because there will often be a greater degree of approximation involved in their compilation. Furthermore they will not necessarily be available to all readers of the final report of the dietary study.

Sometimes it is useful to create many new and detailed codes to help inexperienced coders, even though the new codes may be given very similar, or even identical nutrient values, to related foods in the basic table. This system also allows more detailed subdivision into food groups or ingredients (9.2.4). It also keeps the future options open if subsequently more composition information becomes available for the particular food item or for calculation of a wider range of nutrients.

8.3.7. Nutrients not listed in tables

It is rarely possible to give a value for every nutrient in every food in food tables. However, many of the gaps are confined to less important nutrients in foods used less frequently. For example, the intake of minor B vitamins may be underestimated by some 1–14 per cent using the McCance and Widdowson fourth edition.[5,17] This problem will not be encountered for energy, protein, fat, or carbohydrate, and not usually for iron, calcium, thiamin, riboflavin, nicotinic acid, or vitamin C. Other nutrients will have varying degrees of missing values and any study of such nutrients should ensure that appropriate values are found. Calculation of the frequency of consumption of all the foods in the study is also necessary to establish whether any missing values are associated with important foods.

For nutrients not listed in the tables at all, a new table must be compiled either from the literature or analytical sources. Useful values for selected foods, for example, are tabulated in the recently published fourteenth edition of Bowes and Church's tables[19] for chromium, cobalt, fluoride, iodine, molybdenum, nickel, selenium, tin, vitamin K, caffeine, choline, myo-inositol, nitrite, nitrate, oxalic acid, phytic acid, phytosterol, saccharin, and theobromine.

8.4. Databases

8.4.1. International bases

With the increasing use of computers in dietary calculations and the general accumulation of published work on food composition, large scale food or nutrient databases are being created by national and international organizations. The aim of these is to provide a comprehensive and readily accessible source of nutrient values in foods. This source is often more detailed and up to date than other food composition tables published relatively infrequently. These activities are being directed by the international organization INFOODS (International Network of Food Data Systems)[20] based on regional continental organizations such as EUROFOODS[26] and ASIAFOODS, and others are being formed, such as LATINFOODS, AFRICAFOODS, and MENAFOODS (Middle East and North Africa). The aims of INFOODS are:

(1) to collate and coordinate existing data on food composition tables;

(2) to make recommendations for data quality;[12]

(3) to set up an international terminology and nomenclature system;

(4) to provide a firm base for exchange of information between users and their needs.

In addition to these general aims, EUROFOODS have also set up an active computer group in which national European tables are being merged into one database, designed for use in a wide variety of situations. A forerunner to these schemes is the US Department of Agriculture which has had a nutrient data bank in existence for some years.[16]

8.4.2. Comparisons between databases

Comparisons between computerized databases are merely a sophisticated reflection of the differences in the food composition tables from which the bases are derived. The sources of variability are therefore essentially the same as have been described for the tables themselves (8.2). Comparative studies between databases will also reflect individual interpretation on coding of foods and whether this is done manually or by computer.

Some variability may also arise between different modified and shortened systems, even though they are based on the same primary food composition table. In general, greater compatibility can be expected for mean intakes of energy, protein, fat, minerals such as potassium and phosphorus, and some B vitamins, for example, B_6 and B_{12}. For most of the other nutrients, results have shown greater variability between databases.[1,4,23]

Some examples are illustrated in Table 8.4.

It is important to recognize that all these different calculated values are themselves estimates of the actual composition of the dietary mixture. In view of the remarks made earlier about the accuracy of food composition tables, the agreement is quite good. Table 8.4 illustrates the common and incorrect implication of the accuracy of these calculations. The energy values are based on assumptions that are known to be extremely limited (accuracies of 1 in 5000–7000 kJ (1195–1675 kcal)) using factors that have at the most three significant figures. Likewise, calcium values are expressed to 1 part in 800 which far exceeds the analytical precision of the method. It is therefore most important that those who are responsible for interpreting the nutritional analysis obtained from databases should be thoroughly familiar with the food composition table from which the database is derived. With the rapidly increasing availability of individual and commercial systems, merely to send off food records for analysis and use the subsequent results uncritically, is a pitfall which must be avoided.

8.4.3. Practical use of computer databases

Food composition tables contain large amounts of data, and they need to be readily and quickly accessed. Often calculations using these data tend to be repetitive and are, therefore, subject to errors. These three points alone make such tables a priority for storage in computers. However,

Table 8.4. Examples of daily energy and nutrient intakes calculated using different nutrient databases with three sets of food intake records

	Energy* kcal	Energy* kJ	Protein g	Fat g	Ca mg	Fe mg	Vit C mg
Arab 1985†							
A	1070	4,455	48	50	172	6.2	34
B	1140	4,757	43	55	181	10.0	55
C	1200	5,003	54	65	406	6.3	50
D	1250	5,227	54	67	384	6.5	44
E	1280	5,354	55	69	295	6.8	40
F	1300	5,443	40	71	225	8.8	49
G	1470	6,163	66	70	111	4.7	46
Bagu and Rutishauser, 1984‡							
SODA 1	1790	7,481	65.2	81.6	775	10.9	125
NUTRITION	1700	7,090	65.7	78.1	834	10.3	104
APPLE	1770	7,415	71.4	71.4	822	14.1	145
Taylor *et al.*, 1985§							
A	1706	**7,140**	75	72	1088	10.9	89
B	1660	**6,950**	72	70	966	14.2	103
C	1680	**7,030**	74	73	1023	9.7	93

*As the authors did not give both kcal and kJ, values in italics (here written in boldface type) have been calculated from the mean results presented using the factor 1 kcal = 4.184 kJ.
†One 2-day dietary protocol calculated by seven European Research Centres.
‡Eighteen 14-day dietary records calculated using W. Australian (SODA), British (NUTRITION), and US (APPLE) databases.
§Twenty-four 1-day dietary records calculated using three US databases.

some thought is required as to what data are to be recorded, how they are to be stored and what software will be required to use them.

8.5. Setting up a computer database

The forms in which computer-readable food composition tables are provided can cause problems when loading the data into a computer. For example, when the fourth edition of the McCance and Widdowson table[17] was published, it was made available simultaneously as a series of punched paper tapes. These were bulky and presented some difficulties when they came to be read. There were variations in what information was recorded for a food, depending on its food group. There were 30 values which were common to all foods—energy, protein, fat, carbohydrate, minerals, and vitamins, and, in addition, there were others which were only present in foods within one or two food groups. For example, lactose was only to be found in milk and milk foods. Such variations can cause problems at the programming stage and it is recommended that such variations be removed at the earliest opportunity during the storing of the database. One way to achieve this is to make certain that every food has a value for every component. For example, all foods would have a value for lactose, even though in the majority of foods this value would be zero. These variations in data format are not peculiar to paper tape. They may be met whatever the recording medium.

Databases recorded on magnetic tapes are less bulky, but they are not free of problems. The difficulties with this medium lie in the format used to record data. Large main-frame computers are usually able to handle a variety of tape formats and so present less of a problem. Many mini-computer installations do not have facilities for reading reels of magnetic tape, but with the inter-connection of computers becoming more and more common (by telephone, for example) it is comparatively easy to read a magnetic tape on one machine and transfer its contents to another.

With the increasing availability of micro-computers all of which seem to have floppy disk drive units, the problems become very serious because there is, as yet, no common standard for recording data on to such disks. This makes it impossible to transfer data from the machine of one manufacturer to that of another. Again, however, the transfer of data from a large machine to one of the user's choice is becoming increasingly common.

A major consideration in establishing a computerized food composition table is the size of the table and how much room is available on the mass storage devices such as disks or magnetic tape. It is to be assumed that a working copy of the database would be recorded on to a disk as this provides a file which may be accessed randomly, whereas a tape may only be read sequentially and is, therefore, much slower to use.

As an example to find out approximately how much storage space is required, consider the McCance and Widdowson tables. In the fourth edition records are found for about 970 foods. Using the basic table, but ignoring cholesterol, fatty acids, and amino acids, there are 39 values for each food, plus a code for the food group and the food's code number, giving a total of 41 numbers. If each value is recorded as a 'real' number, that is with decimal parts, each value will occupy at least 4 bytes of storage, so that the full table would require some 151 320 bytes. Integers (whole numbers) can take only 2 bytes, reducing the required storage space to 75 660 bytes. If, in addition, cholesterol and fatty acids were also to be recorded, another 82 bytes per food would be used, giving an overall need for 155 200 bytes. In each case, these figures may be regarded as minimal because the calculations do not take into account either the space required for the recording of the food names, or the space which would be needed, if and when extra foods are added to the database.

With main-frames and mini-computers, this space requirement may not be a serious problem, but with micromachines a compromise must be reached. One solution would be to have the full table on one or two floppy disks and to have a program which would run through the full file to abstract those components of interest to the user and record them on to a separate working disk.

How can these data be stored as integers when the majority are expressed as 'reals' to one, two, or even three places of decimals?

Each must be multiplied by a factor specific to each component so that integers may be produced with no loss of precision. This process has disadvantages because there may be a limit to the maximum size of an integer. A 16-bit computer, that is one whose word length is 16 bits, will have a maximum integer of 32 767. Any value above this number will produce a negative quantity and if more than twice the limit, it will become positive again! There may well be occasions when this limit is exceeded.

Take, for example, the values for vitamin D in the McCance and Widdowson table, which are expressed to three decimal places. The multiplier used must, therefore, be 1000. However, with cod liver oil, the stated level of vitamin D is 210 μg/100 g, and this multiplied by 1000 gives 210 000. The computer will arrive at a final value of 13 392. One way to overcome this difficulty is to make such cases negative and then divide by 10. This would give a final value of $-21 000$. Of course, such manipulation may involve the loss of some precision. In the worst case, this would be 8 in 32 768, or 0.024 per cent, an acceptable loss, considering the variability inherent in the composition of foods (8.2.2 and 8.2.4).

This discussion of storage space required has, so far, been confined to requirements within the mass storage devices. How much space will be required for the software which must be written to use the database? Will it be possible to store some of the database information in memory to reduce the time used searching for data?

Unfortunately, it is not possible to answer the first question because so many imponderables are involved—including what is the application, how many nutrients will be involved, how complex will the program be? Because there can be no direct answer to this first question, neither can there be one to the second. It would depend on both the first answer and the size of the computer's memory. In an ideal situation the whole of the database would be read into the machine's memory. This could be done on a main-frame, but with smaller machines it would not be possible, and a compromise would have to be made.

It has been shown that most people eat a relatively small number of foods[7]. Figure 8.3 shows how relatively small numbers of foods make up a large proportion of dietary consumption, with 200 foods accounting for just over 90 per cent of all foods eaten during one large survey.

If there is sufficient room within the computer's memory to hold the

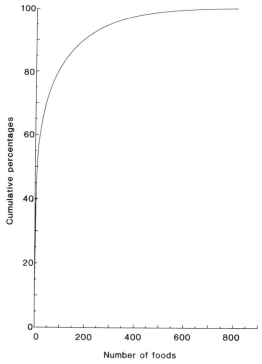

Fig. 8.3. Number and frequency of foods occurring in the diets of Cambridge women studied by Black *et al.*[5]

data for these 200 most commonly eaten foods, then the saving in time during calculations would be considerable. Even if only a few foods could be stored in this way, the saving would be worth while.

8.5.1. Missing values and traces

As mentioned earlier (8.2.2) there are foods for which no information is available for one or more components, as shown by a dash, (—), and there are other components which are reported as traces. These should be distinguishable from zero within the database because they are, in all probability, not zero.

When it comes to calculating intakes, how should the programmer treat them? Unfortunately, there is little that can be done *except* to take them as zero or assign a value from another source.

A similar dilemma occurs when ranges for values have been stored in the database. Which should be used? The maximum, the minimum, some arbitrary value between or *the value*?

Unless the programmer is willing, or able to write some complex software to take all possible circumstances into account, it will be *the value* which is used.

This is why results produced by computers should not be regarded as having been handed down on tablets of stone, but should be taken with a large pinch of salt!

8.6. Creation of a limited file for a specific community study

In spite of the increasing availability of food composition data, there are still many situations where dietary investigations are made and there is no information on the composition of the foods, particularly the local cooked items. If the investigators are fortunate enough to possess, or have access to laboratory facilities, it is possible to start at the beginning of the study by constructing one's own nutrient database. Such a system has been developed, for example, for the computer analysis of the food consumption records obtained in a study in the Gambia (6.3.2 and 13.4.4).

References

1. Arab, L. (1985). Summary of Survey of Food Composition Tables and Nutrient Data Banks in Europe. In: *EUROFOODS: Towards Compatibility of Nutrient Data Banks in Europe. Ann. Nutr. Metab.* (Suppl. 1) **29**, 39–45.
2. Arab, L. and Wittler, M. (1985). *European Food Composition Tables:*

Introductory Materials in Translation. A EUROFOODS Computer Committee Project.

3. Arab, L. and Wittler, M. (1985). *European Food Composition Tables: Comparison of Modes of Expression.* A EUROFOODS Computer Committee Project.
4. Bagu, K. and Rutishauser, I. H. E. (1984). Comparison of computerized nutrient analysis programs based on Australian, British and American tables of food composition. *J. Food Nutr.* **41**, 17–20.
5. Black, A. E., Paul, A. A., and Hall, C. (1985). Footnotes to food tables 2. The underestimations of intakes of lesser B vitamins by pregnant and lactating women as calculated using the fourth edition of McCance and Widdowson's *The Composition of Foods. Hum. Nutr. Appl. Nutr.* **39A**, 19–22.
6. Day, K. C. (1980). 'Recipe', a computer program for calculating the nutrient contents of foods. *J. Hum. Nutr.* **34**, 181–7.
7. Day, K. C. (1985). Nutrient data banks from the point of view of the computer programmer. In: *EUROFOODS: Towards compatibility of nutrient data banks. Ann. Nutr. Metab.* (Suppl. 1) **29**, 54–9.
8. FAO (1975). *Food composition tables, updated annotated bibliography.* Nutrition Policy and Programmes Service. FAO, Rome.
9. FAO, USDA (1982). Food composition tables for the near East. *FAO Food and Nutrition Paper No. 26.* FAO, Rome.
10. FAO/WHO (1973). Energy and protein requirements. *WHO Tech. Rep. Ser. No. 522.* WHO, Geneva.
11. FAO/WHO/UNU (1985). Energy and Protein Requirements. *WHO Tech. Rep. Ser. No. 724.* WHO, Geneva.
12. Greenfield, H. and Southgate, D. A. T. (1985). A pragmatic approach to the production of good quality food composition data. *ASEAN Food J.* **1**, 47–54.
13. INFOODS (1986). *International directory of food composition tables.* International Network of Food Data Systems Secretariat. Massachusetts Institute of Technology, Cambridge, Massachusetts.
14. International Union of Nutritional Sciences Committee 1/1, Nomenclature (1978). Genetic descriptor and trivial names for vitamins and related compounds. *Recomm. Nutr. Abst. Rev.* **48**, 831–5.
15. Merrill, A. L. and Watt, B. K. (1955). Energy value of foods—basis and derivation. *USDA Agric. Handbook No. 74.* Washington, DC.
16. Murphy, E. W., Watt, B. K., and Rizek, R. L. (1974). US Department of Agriculture Nutrient Data Bank. *J. Assoc. Off. Anal. Chem.* **57**, 1198–204.
17. Paul, A. A. and Southgate, D. A. T. (1978). In: McCance, R. A. and Widdowson, E. M. *The composition of foods* (4th revised edition). HMSO, London.
18. Paul, A. A., Southgate, D. A. T., and Buss, D. H. (1986). In: *The composition of foods*: supplementary information and review of new compositional data. (ed. R. A. McCance and E. M. Widdowson). *Hum. Nutr. Appl. Nutr.* **40A**, 287–99.
19. Pennington, J. A. T. and Church, H. N. (1985). *Bowes and Church's food values of portions commonly used.* (14th edition), J. B. Lippincott, Philadelphia.

20. Rand, W. M. and Young, V. R. (1983). International Network of Food Data Systems (INFOODS): report of a small international planning conference. *Food Nutr. Bull.* **5**, 15–23.
21. Royal Society (1972). Metric units, conversion factors, and nomenclature in nutritional and food sciences. Report of the Subcommittee for Nutritional Sciences.
22. Southgate, D. A. T. (1983). Availability of and needs for reliable analytical methods for the assay of foods. *Food Nutr. Bull.* **5**, 30–9.
23. Taylor, M. L., Kozlowski, B. W., and Baer, M. T. (1985). Energy and nutrient values from different computerized data basis. *J. Am. Diet Assoc.* **85**, 1136–8.
24. Thomas, S. and Corden, M. (1977). *Tables of composition of Australian foods.* Revised edition. Australian Commonwealth Department of Health, Canberra.
25. US Department of Agriculture (1976–86). Composition of foods, raw, processed, prepared. *Agriculture Handbook No. 8.1 to 8.14.* USDA, Washington, DC.
26. West, C. E. (1985). EUROFOODS: towards compatibility of nutrient data banks in Europe. *Ann. Nutr. Metab.* (Suppl. 1) **29**, 1–72.
27. Widdowson, E. M. (1978). Note on the calculation of the energy value of foods and diets. In: McCance, R. A. and Widdowson, E. M. *The composition of foods* (4th edition) (Paul, A. A. and Southgate, D. A. T., eds). HMSO, London.
28. Widdowson, E. M. and McCance, R. A. (1943). Food tables, their scope and limitations. *Lancet* **ii**, 230–2.
29. Wu Leung, W. T., Busson, F., and Jardin, C. (1968). *Food composition table for use in Africa.* US Department of Health, Education, and Welfare, National Center for Chronic Disease Control, Bethesda, MD, and Nutrition Division, FAO, Rome.
30. Wu Leung, W. T., Butrum, R. R., and Chang, F. H. (1972). *Food composition table for use in Asia.* US Department of Health, Education, and Welfare, National Institute of Arthritis, Metabolism, and Digestive Diseases, Bethesda, MD, and FAO, Rome.
31. Wu Leung, W. T. and Flores, M. (1961). *INCAP–ICNND food composition table for use in Latin America.* National Institute of Health, Bethesda, MD, and INCAP, Guatemala City, Mexico.

9

Analyses, presentation, and interpretation of results

LENORE ARAB

Introduction

Many scientists conducting nutritional studies invest tremendous efforts in collecting detailed, accurate, and extensive information on food consumption behaviour. They are then surprised to discover that after completing the field work the job is only half over and the real difficulties have begun. If there is no access to previously developed and tested programs for collection, coding, and quality control of information on types and amounts of foods eaten, preparation losses, and waste, the total job can be immense. The lack of an available, appropriate coding system for converting the food description into machine readable form is often an unpleasant discovery. This chapter attempts to prepare the reader for the range of tasks involved in the analyses, presentation, and interpretation of results.

It goes without saying that the data analyses and presentation is entirely dependent upon the purposes of the study and its resulting design. However, the range of food consumption survey aims is such that they can be grouped in a few broad categories for discussion (Chapters 4 and 6).

The complexity of analysis and interpretation is increased by the uncontrolled variations in dietary assessment methods and the range of dimensions of food consumption. In the simplest study, yes or no questions can be asked to determine whether or not person x eats food y. The next level of complexity is analysis by category of frequency of intake of specific foods or food groups ('many times a day, week or month, or seldom'). A further level is the quantitative study of foods consumed and the level of daily nutrient intakes (or confidence intervals). Finally where, when and how preserved, prepared, packaged foods have been consumed.

The development of a complex database for storing the individual information is required for numerous types of analyses. Discussion of data analysis begins with the data handling steps. It includes database design, summarized statistical analyses, presentation formats and finally the critical interpretation of the results as based on the strengths and weaknesses of the study and the variability, biases and error of measurement.

9.1. Data analyses

The various aims of nutrition surveys are outlined in Chapter 4, and the different types of information to be collected for these aims are described in Chapter 6. Even if the study attempts to do no more than determine group level intakes (type 1 information), individual data need to be processed and totalled. The data handling steps generally include:

(1) data collection and coding;

(2) entry into a computer base;

(3) validating the entered data against the original documents and acceptable ranges;

(4) calculation of nutrient intakes.

Figure 9.1 summarizes these steps which are discussed in detail in the following section.

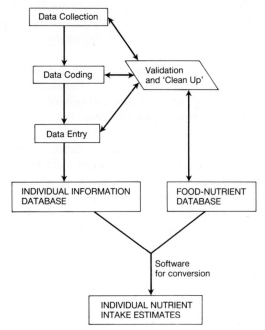

Fig. 9.1. Data handling procedures.

9.1.1. Data collection

The actual questions about, or records of dietary behaviour are the basis of data collections. Methodology for this has been discussed in Chapters 5 and 6 and involves all aspects, from interviewer training and proper questioning to the keeping of clear, exact, and detailed schedules and records. Mention should be made of the ability to computerize data collection or dietary interviews. This can eliminate manual efforts in the next three areas of coding, entry, and validation.[2,3]

9.1.2. Data coding

Data coding is the conversion of the collected information into clearly defined machine readable form. There are tens of thousands of products available for consumption at supermarkets around the world. International comparisons depend on similar coding and grouping schemes as well as standardized coding rules for what goes into which food group.

The coding system used should preserve detailed information as well as providing the sum totals. It should be emphasized that the use of different coding schemes and coding rules hinder comparisons between studies. Often even with the best of intentions in 'cross coding' there is frustration because of practical difficulties in separating out individual food items from groups or finding a satisfactory common denominator. Such problems are illustrated in Fig. 9.2.

The example shows two different coding schemes. True cross coding is not possible in either the case of code 1 to 2 or for code 2 to 1. Conversion of code 1 to 2 is only possible for the third group, 'EF', which would belong to group 3 in code 2. For all other code 1 food groups, no direct cross-over coding is possible. For group 1 of code 1, part would belong in group 1 of code 2 and part in group 2, but once coded together they are no longer separable and the information on individual food items is lost. For accurate recording the original records would then be needed. Conversion of code 2 to code 1 is possible only for groups 4 and 5; G and H would be coded GH. DEF is irreversibly combined, and cannot be entered into groups CD and EF.

These arguments support the selection and use of an appropriate standard food code to allow cross comparisons between studies.

Traditionally, coding has been done manually with a person searching for the proper code from food tables and transferring it to survey schedules with the subject's identity code, data, meal, food code, processing code, and amount codes.

Despite the problems involved, conversion of foods reported eaten into standard, clearly described machine readable form is a necessary step in dietary assessment. Only very limited questionnaires can offer pre-coded formats.

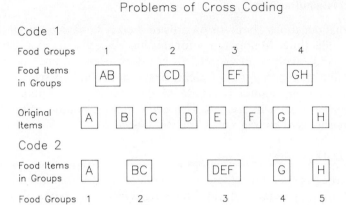

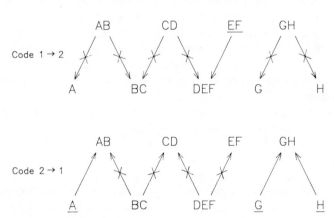

Fig. 9.2. Problems of cross-coding.

The basic requirements for coding intakes are usually in a manual for code design and coding guidelines along with a handbook with computer entry systems. Included in the requirements are:

(1) alphabetical list of foods, including synonyms, which individually itemizes all foods of interest;

(2) numerical code list with food names and code numbers;

(3) coding procedures to follow when an incomplete food description is given;

(4) list of foods, not in the coding system, with their weights, portion sizes, or complete descriptions, and instructions for the code under which they should be classified;

(5) schedules or record forms on which coding problems and the coder's impromptu decisions can be recorded;

(6) list of normal portion sizes of individual food items;

(7) a table to convert household measures of individual foods into grams weight;

(8) short list of emergency advice and procedures (Save data);

(9) correction guidelines for wrongly entered information;

(10) list of telephone numbers for emergency aid: systems level, software level, coding problems, and general.

Unforeseen problems always arise during coding and it is rare that a code is complete with all the foods eaten.

Good communications are therefore necessary between the coder and principle fieldworkers and also with someone capable of making nutritionally relevant coding decisions when such problems appear.

9.1.3. Data entry and validation

Generally, the coded information is either entered on-line or off-line into a computer system, leaving open the potential for transcription errors. A number of strategies to prevent this are feasible. One is to present the original text with the code. Another is to ensure that entry personnel print and compare their work before storing it.

These efforts can be supplemented by the inclusion of programs which check the amounts of the foods entered and compare them with previously agreed plausibility ranges. This can be done at the same time so that any suspicious values initiate an immediate response or query to the entry personnel. Typical plausibility ranges include maximal absolute amounts consumed per person per day and maximal and minimal portion sizes for individual foods. This, depending on the size of the food code, can require considerable storage space.

9.1.4. Database design

Once the information has been coded, entered, checked, validated, and confirmed, it is advisable to read it into a database for manipulation of the foods and amounts as well as the calculation of the energy and nutrients consumed. The design of this database depends on the available software. This design is also a function of the level of information to be maintained. The inherent hierarchical structure of food intake information over a week is shown in Fig. 9.3.

Consideration should be given at the start of the study to the parameters of interest, the level of the exactness, the frequencies of consumptions, codes and the relationships to be stored. Careful thought and

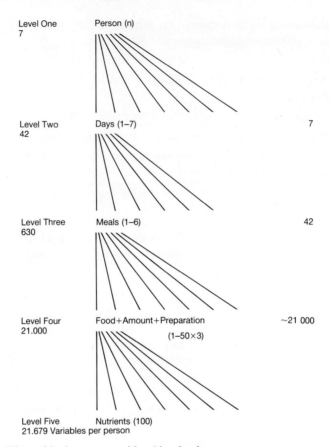

Fig. 9.3. Hierarchical structure of food intake data.

planning are necessary to ensure availability of all desired information in a usable form. Generally the minimum information to be handled is food code, preparation code, waste amount per meal, and food per person, per day (Fig. 9.3). Further expansion of this information base would be needed to allow for selected structures and relationships as they exist in recipes; combinations of foods, proportions, and preparation methods.

Database design also includes the hardware and software components. For handling large sets of food consumption data a computer is strongly recommended. Storage requirements will range from 10 to 500 variables per subject depending on the method and extent of the study. For a study of 100 persons, their usual diet and basic socio-economic description, a storage area should be foreseen, independent of the food nutrient database of at least 2 Megabytes; increasing linearly with the number of subjects (8.5).

9.1.5. Data clean-up (validation)

Even the most carefully handled dataset can rarely be converted into machine readable form without human error.

Typical errors include:

(1) reading and/or transcription errors;
(2) wrong or improbable amounts;
(3) numerical inversions of digits, resulting in wrong codes or amounts;
(4) amounts or codes being entered twice;
(5) inversion of amount and code so that the code is taken as the amount and *vice versa*.

More extensive errors occur when:

(1) parts of meals, entire meals or entire days are overlooked by the coder, or coded twice;
(2) wrong identification numbers are assigned to subjects and entered;
(3) data are accidentally read twice into the database, resulting in doubled amounts per day;
(4) sequences of data are shifted so that entire data lines are misread;
(5) segments of the data are accidentally lost or erased or found unreadable once in the computer system.

Owing to the range of expected and possible errors, the quality of the data needs to be checked in all the areas where problems may arise (that is, all manual and some automated processes). Proper quality control requires that complete spot checks are made of sub-samples of the stored data against the original documents. This should be undertaken to various degrees at various stages and certainly after all the handling has been completed and the final database is established.

In addition to this, frequency distributions for all food codes and all amounts for each food code should be made over the entire dataset and examined by someone experienced with the dietary behaviour of the population being studied. At this step implausible amounts and unacceptable codes can be identified, using a printout of the subject's identification, day, meal item, and amount, against the original records. If an error is detected, it is wise to examine printouts for the entire day surrounding the error for any other possible discrepancies. It could happen that an entire data line is shifted upon input and that for a given subsection of data, all amounts and codes are incorrect.

Increasingly, personal computer-based programs are being developed to combine the coding and entry steps, thus saving time, eliminating many sources of transcription errors and incorporating editing and error checking routines at this work step.[4,8]

Information (Files)

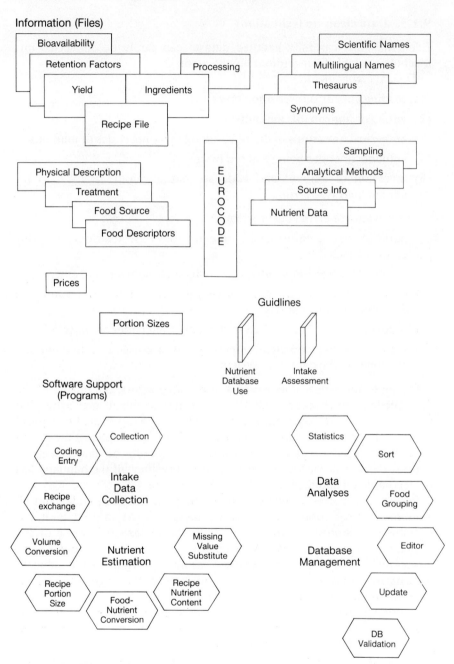

Fig. 9.4. Components of an extensive dietary assessment system.
Source: Arab.[4]

The sophisticated user of food and nutrient information wants data including nutrient content per 100 g or 1 kg of food, nutrient changes due to preparation, and bioavailability, to calculate the best possible estimates of nutrient intake per person. All components of a theoretical system, both information files (data sets) and software for use can be seen in Fig. 9.4.

These data sets, as far as available, also need to be checked for completeness and correctness. This, for example, can take the form of checks on the range of specific nutrients per food group based on wet or dry weight, or on the fat or non-fat content.

A printout of all coded consumed foods for which incomplete or no nutrient intake information is available will help to anticipate invalid coded and incomplete nutrient databases. Invalid codes can be corrected by linking the information to an individual, day and meal; and validating its correctness in the context of that meal. Missing nutrient information in the food composition database is a real problem requiring a great deal of effort to solve. Advice for handling these problems is scanty and beyond the scope of this chapter.

The step after food to nutrient conversion, should be the production of a frequency distribution of absolute energy intakes per day for the population and examination to see if the extreme values, both high and low, reflect the original dietary protocol of these individuals. Similarly, frequency distributions for number of codes per person, number of meals per person and number of days per person should be produced and examined for irregularities.

9.1.6. Estimation of nutrient intakes from food consumption records

Besides the individual consumption data, a food–nutrient database is required for conversion of this information to estimates of individual daily nutrient intakes as seen in Fig. 9.1. This second database, regardless of its source, needs to be checked by the user for completeness, in terms of its range of foods and their processed forms, as well as for missing nutrient values for individual foods. As mentioned (9.1.5), values are required for all nutrients of interest for all foods coded and of significance to the study. Inevitably problems arise either because foods are consumed and they do not appear in the tables or there are numerous nutrient values missing. Programs are also needed to convert food intakes into nutrient intake estimations. Nutrient intake estimates should, for a number of reasons outlined in Table 9.1, be considered with caution to accurately represent the usual short-term or constant levels of individual nutrient intake. Estimation of nutrient intakes is discussed in detail in Chapter 8.

Table 9.1. Nutrient intake analyses from dietary records; reasons why they are not accurate estimates of short term or usual intakes

1. Not all foods eaten might be reported and *vice versa.*
2. Some information could be so badly recorded that it is unusable.
3. Actual amounts consumed are almost impossible to determine because of faulty estimation of size, non-measurements of waste (bone, skin, pips etc.), different water contents (e.g. of noodles), uptake of fats and spices in cooking, loss of water, ice cubes in drinks, and the like. Estimates can be more than 100 per cent inaccurate.
4. Absorption and use of nutrients differ. A result of illness, medications and foods eaten together at a meal may enhance or inhibit absorption.
5. Food table values are averages from a variety of samples, none of which was the food actually consumed.
6. Most food tables have many missing values.
7. Many foods eaten are not listed in one set of food tables or they may only be part of the average for a food group.
8. The period of the survey reported might be a poor reflection of the individuals usual intakes or may have been biased by observation effects.

Adapted from Arab.[2]

9.1.7. Application of computers

Increasing storage and speed capacities, reduced costs and the wide-spread development of software for various purposes are making personal computers more and more attractive for direct and intense application in dietary assessment studies. The benefits of increased automation of dietary assessment include:

(1) reduced cost of data collection;
(2) potential for more detailed and standardized interviewing;
(3) fewer errors due to reduction in data handling steps;
(4) the speed of results (immediate); and
(5) the potential for supplying the subject an evaluation of his or her dietary behaviour.

The advantages of full automation are:
(1) no between interviewer variability (standardization);
(2) no response bias induced by interviewer (non-objectivity);
(3) no change in dietary behaviour induced by the method of assessment;

(4) the scientist decides on exact phrasing, depth of probe, and sequences of questioning;

(5) no hand coding of food information into machine as needed before;

(6) built in and immediate editing and checking (validation) routines (automated quality control);

(7) immediate results;

(8) better comparability of results;

(9) reduced costs of collecting and assessing dietary information.

The current experience in application is presented elsewhere.[2,3,8]

Although few programs are available for collection of dietary information, many are on the market which allow for calculations from intake information or recipes, and include their own food composition database.[13] They vary in their range of capabilities, required hardware, extent of nutrient database, (number of foods, nutrients and missing values), and expense.

A later stage of dietary assessment is the statistical analysis and presentation of results. Software packages, not designed for, but readily applicable to food assessment study needs, are available. Some of the most commonly used are SAS[16] and SPSS.[17]

These, and numerous other programs are available for main-frame computers and more recently, at least in more simplified versions, for IBM compatible personal computers. These programs and others (for example PLOT-IT[11]) can also eliminate the need for hand-made graphic data presentations.

Major advances are taking place which should revolutionize dietary assessment. However, at present the pioneering phase is still underway. There are numerous dangers and considerations in deciding how far, and in which areas, the nutritionist should develop and become dependent on computers for study results. Certainly price, availability of hardware and software, and their servicing are a few. Language is another important consideration, especially since access is often not provided to code programs and therefore no alterations in the acquired software can be made.

Compatibility of software programs for different purposes, one to another and to different machines is also an issue worthy of careful consideration.

The nutritionists and computer specialists would be well advised to allow development and support of the computerized system to be a joint effort.

Finally, automated field work involves the risk of break down, power loss, diskette destruction, or theft. Therefore defensive lines of 'back-up' need to be anticipated for such contingencies.

9.1.8. Statistical analyses

Summarization of results, comparisons of groups, identification of inter-relationships and hypotheses testing will almost certainly require statistical analyses of the collected and validated dietary data. Due to the widespread availability of statistical packages which have been subjected to years of experience, testing, and validation, it is not recommended that investigators begin programming statistical procedures. Many hand held calculators are pre-programmed to provide means, variances, standard deviations, correlation coefficients and regression coefficients. However, it is still better to use standard software packages compatible with the database as it is stored. Two commonly used packages not specially developed for nutritional or medical use, but readily applicable for these needs have been mentioned earlier.[16, 17]

In the following section recommendations for appropriate statistics for different purposes of presentation and analyses are made. The use of statistical procedures for taking confounding effects, variability and biases into account are discussed in 9.3.

9.2. Presentation

An effective presentation of results is based on the purpose of the study of analyses, the target group for whom the presentation is intended, and the information that is wanted as a basis for discussion. In general, information from dietary assessment is presented as descriptions of central tendencies, distributions of intake, or as inter-relationships between dietary intakes and continuously measured parameters such as indicators of health risk, for example, serum cholesterol, blood pressure, or urinary parameters. These are compared with eating behaviours between groups of individuals such as in case control studies or in socio-economic comparisons. This section will suggest various presentation forms and present a discussion of the basis of comparison in dietary studies and the more generally applied units of measurement of dietary behaviour.

9.2.1. Measurement of central tendencies

Databases, as described earlier in this chapter require manipulation to convert the given information into a suitable form for descriptive scientific purposes and analytical procedures. For each nutrient of interest, and for foods as well, summary statistics for the group of individuals of interest are uesful. This can be expressed as the group average, which is the sum of the nutrient amount consumed divided by the number of persons assessed and expressed either as a daily, weekly, or meal event.

$$\bar{x} = \frac{\Sigma/x}{n}.$$

The median, or the middle measurement, is generally more useful for reviewing intake levels of a group or population as a whole. This is because a few individuals, with excess of intake, can cause an average intake to be actually greater than that consumed by most of the individuals assessed. The median is derived by listing all scores sequentially and, if the total is an odd number, taking the middle score. If it is an even number, the half-way point between the two values surrounding the middle is taken.

In addition to the mean or median, as summary statistic for central tendency (locality), the standard deviation may be reported as a summary statistic for variability (spread) among the individuals in a group or population. The standard deviation (SD) is the square root of the variance of a distribution and is an index of variability in the original measurement units. It is calculated from the observations in a group as:

$$SD = \sqrt{\frac{\Sigma(x - \bar{x})^2}{n - 1}}$$

A coefficient of variation (CV) is a standardized measure of spread offering comparability between different units of measure. It is calculated by dividing the standard deviation by the mean and generally it is expressed as a percentage:

$$CV = \frac{SD}{\bar{x}} \times 100\%$$

For summarizing non-normal distributions, percentiles (P_{10}, P_{25} etc) or ranges are more appropriate to indicate variability.

To account for sampling error in the estimation of the mean when sample sizes are small or moderate, standard errors of the mean or confidence intervals are commonly reported. The standard error (SE) is a measure of the accuracy of the sample mean ($\bar{x}$) as an estimation of the population mean. It is incidentally, calculated from the standard deviation and the sample size (n):

$$SE = SD/\sqrt{n}.$$

Confidence limits indicate the interval in which the true (population) mean is likely to be situated. For instance, when n is reasonably large, approximate 90 per cent confidence limits are calculated as:

$$CL = \bar{x} \pm 1.65\,(SE).$$

9.2.2. Distributions

Presentation of the entire population distribution of intake of a given nutrient or food is much more useful for the scientist or health planner than a single point value such as the mean or median. In a distribution of the population, extremes are visible and the size of the population can be readily interpreted from it (Fig. 9.5). If, however, software is not available for preparing this automatically, it can be a very time consuming exercise. Though figures make a stronger impact than tables, they also require much more space in a text. They are therefore inappropriate for presenting distributions of numerous parameters.

The histogram is a familiar figure to illustrate distributions. It also has the advantage that normality of distribution and skewedness are readily visible. The disadvantage is that this distribution does not allow visual interpolation of the percentage of individuals at risk at different cut-off points. In addition, the median is not obvious to see.

By contrast, a cumulative percentage distribution of intake, allows the reader to select any percentile of interest or any level of intake of interest

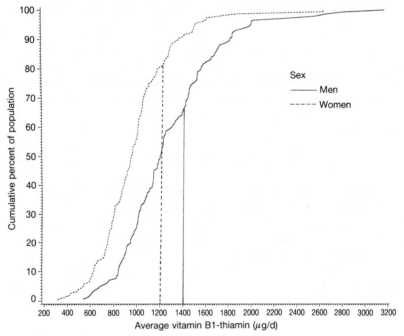

Fig. 9.5. Cumulative percentage distribution of thiamin intakes (μg/day) in spring 1982.

———— men (n=1153)
– – – – women (n=1183)

Source: Arab *et al.*[6]

and see what the corresponding values for this population were. Cumulative percentage distributions can be drawn rapidly by hand. To do this, with the *y*-axis representing the percentile and the *x*-axis the levels of intake, the following percentile can be read from a frequency list, plotted, and a smoothed curve drawn between (Fig. 9.5). Recommended percentiles are 0.5, 1.0, 2.5, 5.0, 10, 20, 40, 50, 60, 80, 90, 95, 97.5, 99, 99.5, and 100.

9.2.3. Presentation of group comparisons

Four different approaches, or a combination thereof, can be used to present the intakes in different groups.

The means and standard deviations in the comparison groups can be shown in Table 9.2A.

The result of tests determining the statistical significance of the results for the sample size in question can be reported. The Student's t-tests would be advisable for comparisons of absolute values in the two groups. The medians can also be presented. The Wilcoxon test can be done to test for differences in the two distributions. This provides a non-parametric determination of distribution differences.

If comparisons with recommended levels or assessment of the size of population at risk are desired, it is common to make a presentation in categories of individuals falling into different groups. There might be one in the standard deviation below the recommendations, one between one and two SD below, and another group equalling or exceeding the recommended intake level. For two or more groups this information can be presented in a table and tested for the proportionality of distribution by the chi square test (Table 9.2 B). In the case of most nutrients, it would be even better to apply a probability approach to the population distribution to estimate the size of population at risk, with an intake too high or too low (Table 9.2 C).

Finally, a clear presentation of the differences or similarities between two groups can be made by putting both distributions of intakes in either form suggested above, within the same graph, an example of which can be seen in Fig. 9.5. From this form it can be readily seen if two populations are distinctly different; one higher than the other, if they lie close together or if they cross over. A cross-over might reveal that one population has a specific high-risk group, but otherwise it is similar in its distribution to the other population group.

Out of the multiple criteria which can be applied for dividing the population into groups, the most common analyses are based on comparisons of age, sex, socio-economic status, or different geographical regions. Some other examples include smokers, ex-smokers, passive-smokers, and non-smokers; users of pharmacological agents, for example

Table 9.2. Presentation of group comparisons: intakes of vegetarians and non-vegetarians

2A	Absolute fat intakes (central tendencies)		
	mean g/day	SD	median
Vegetarians (278)	112	17	103
Non-vegetarians (532)	135	24	125
	p=0.05, t-test		
	p=0.03, Wilcoxon test		

2B	Size of risk group in both populations	
	Fat intake	
	< 40%	> 40% of Energy
Vegetarians	113	372
Non-vegetarians	73	436
	$\chi^2 = 13.10; p < 0.001$	

2C	Estimations of real risk group size					
	Average percentage of recommendation consumed		Percentage of persons consuming < 75 per cent of recommendation		Probable percentage of group inadequate	
Nutrients	veg	non-veg	veg	non-veg	veg	non-veg
Vitamin A	287	126	5	12	1	6
Vitamin B$_1$	153	157	15	18	5	6
Vitamin B$_2$	198	105	10	17	7	10
Vitamin C	175	126	18	56	15	40
Vitamin D	56	83	73	48	50	20
Vitamin E	137	95	7	23	6	17

Adapted from Arab.[5]

contraceptives, with non-users or paired comparisons of individuals in different states and time frames; for example, the same individuals at different seasons.

Another approach altogether, is the separation of individuals based upon their nutritional or medical risk status. Commonly, cut-off percentiles are applied and the number of individuals at risk, according to these cut-off percentiles, are presented. Analyses of behavioural differences between the higher-risk and no- or low-risk groups are then carried out.

9.2.4. Units of measure

The purpose of the study and the analyses will be a guide in determining the appropriate units of measure for the question it asks. General population description and group comparisons can be undertaken on the basis of numerous dimensions of dietary behaviour.[4] The measurement is usually done on both the food intake per unit time and the nutrient intake per unit time or per energy content (Table 9.3).

Table 9.3. Units of measure: different ways of expressing results of food consumption studies

Food	Examples
Frequency of consumption	Citrus fruit 5 times/week
	Smoked foods twice/week
Amount per person per day	56 g pork ± 17 g
Nutrients	
Absolute amounts	37 mg vitamin C/day
Nutrient density	1.64 mg/1000 kcal
Percentage of energy	5.6% of energy from alcohol
Nutrient per food source	
Main food contributors of a given nutrient	37% of thiamin from bread
Amount per portion	47% of the daily recommendation from one portion

For foods, the study commonly wants to find out how often they are consumed, what the usual portion sizes are, and what the average or median intake is of the foods, per person, per day.

For nutrients, estimates of the absolute amounts per person per day are most often required, particularly for comparisons with recommended intake levels. The amounts relative to energy intake are also important to estimate adequacy for that level of energy, or to determine whether intakes are too low or nutrient density is poor. Nutrient density expresses the nutrient intake per 4.2 MJ (1000 kcal).

The intakes of the energy sources delivering nutrients are often related to total energy intake by presenting them as a percentage of total energy. For example, a mean intake of 40 g of alcohol may correspond to 7 per cent of total energy intake coming from alcoholic beverages.

9.2.5. Measurements of interrelationships

The examination of interrelationships between dietary parameters and continuous parameters, such as blood pressure, body fat, or serum cholesterol, is often desired (type 3 information). The first consideration to be made here is the expected time-frame of effect. Is a spontaneous relationship being examined, or is an attempt being made to expose the effects of prior dietary behaviour on later status of the dependent parameter (usually a measure of health or an outcome such as disease)?

Case-control studies attempt to look back at behaviour prior to disease. Cohort studies look forward to the events occurring in groups of individuals with distinctly different dietary behaviour. A case-control study is distinctly more difficult from a nutritional point of view.

Regardless of the study design, it is recommended that plots of diet as the independent parameter on the *x*-axis and the dependent parameters of interest on the *y*-axis be constructed as a scattergram. Even if the plots are not used in the final presentation, it is important for the individual responsible for the critical review of this information, to know this way of displaying data as shown in Fig. 9.6. Additional information can be imposed upon the scattergram, in the form of the regression line, of the effect of the independent parameter on the dependent one.

A linearity of effect is assumed here. The true shape of possible relationships, particularly of a dose–response nature, can be better illustrated with smoothing procedure, such as that of Cleveland.[9]

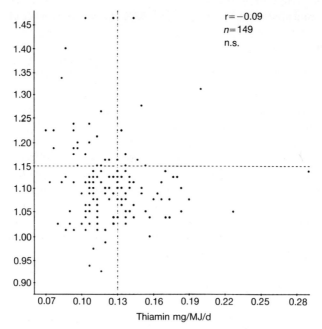

Fig. 9.6. Scattergram of thiamin intakes by erythrocyte transketolase activation levels in young Heidelberg women (*n*=159).
Source: Arab *et al.*[1]

A simple summary description of the relationship can be made through the regression equation itself. Many investigators depend solely on correlation coefficients between the two parameters as a measure of association, even though, if one of the scales has imposed limitations, such as a discrete age range, this can severely distort the result. A thorough discussion of this and the limitations of regression analyses as subject to biological variability, sensitivity, and the population's range of variation is presented by Beaton.[7]

It should be remembered that causality cannot be assumed even with the strongest interrelationship. Sometimes rather misleading results can be found, such as the often found result in cross-sectional surveys, that the energy consumption is inversely related to the body fat. The fatter people eat less.

This phenomena may be due to leaner people being active and consuming more energy. If this is the case (i.e. physical activity is associated with energy intake and, inversely, related to body fat), such a variable is called a confounding factor. The effect of energy consumption on body fat is distorted by the extraneous factor.

Another possible explanation would be a differential bias in reporting food consumption: obese people may underestimate their intake more than others do. This example clearly demonstrates that conclusions cannot be drawn from such cross-sectional interrelationships. The conclusion which would have been drawn here is that eating even more, will make you thinner.

Often the simultaneous analyses of the effect of multiple independent parameters is desired. Generally the aim is either to control for potential confounding factors, or to put into perspective the dietary contributions to a disease state, in relation to other lifestyle, environmental, or genetic factors. Statistical procedures are available to control for external factors and to quantify dietary effects in a contest of multiple determinants of a given outcome. They include multiple linear regression, logistic regression, stratified chi square analyses, and factor and discriminant analyses, to mention a few.

An example of multiple linear regression, applied to determine the effects of dietary factors on HDL cholesterol in a randomly selected population, can be found in Table 9.4. From a number of implicated dietary factors, (energy, animal fat, carbohydrate intakes, plant fat sources, and alcohol intakes), a few explain no variance in the HDL cholesterol of this population. Three dietary factors and six other factors do maintain a significant effect.

The appropriate procedure for controlling confounding and quantifying effects depends largely on the nature of the units of measure and whether they are dichotomous, categorical, or continuous. Selection of a method, its application, and, most importantly, interpretation of the

Table 9.4. Regression analyses* on HDL-cholesterol of young Heidelberg women[1]

Independent parameters	Dependent variable: HDL-cholesterol	
	t values	Regression coefficients
Daily energy/body weight (kcal/kg)	15.65	0.2550
Disaccharide intake (% energy)	20.67	−0.2076
Smoking (number of cigarettes)	17.83	−0.1670
Serum triglycerides (mg/dl)	16.97	−0.1661
Alcohol intake (g/day)	10.05	0.1285
Oral contraceptive use	4.05	−0.0817
Plant fat intake (% of energy)	2.35	−0.0714
Age	2.97	−0.0691
Animal fat (% of energy)	not significant	
Polysaccharides (% of energy)	not significant	

*Stepwise backwards.

findings should be undertaken with the expertise of someone well familiar with the mathematical constraints of the various methods. Both epidemiological and advanced statistical texts offer further details, which are beyond the scope of this manual. They take into account the dimensions of measure of dependent and independent parameters, possible interrelationships and control of confounding in the analyses.[7,9,10]

9.3. Interpretation

A manual for data interpretation, which effectively taught readers to critically evaluate their findings along the way to data interpretation, would be a godsend, and not only in nutritional studies. Unfortunately, good data interpretation also demands knowledge of the study itself, including the validity of the measurements. An appreciation of the constraints involved in converting carefully collected information of foods and amounts into estimations of nutrient intake is also essential. Finally, careful selection of statistical methods is required to ensure that the proper type of statistical test is applied. For example, the appropiate alpha and beta error confidence levels need to be considered so that the results are neither over-interpreted nor non-significant differences or interactions lightly dismissed. Measurement error or sample size or extensive intra-individual variations may, in fact, account for the lack of a statistically significant result.

This section is not an extensive discussion on the above mentioned problems. It rather offers some advice and warns of common failures in data interpretation in nutritional studies.

Too often, dietary surveys are begun and conducted without consideration of data analyses strategy, including an exact phrasing of the questions to be asked of the data, without any conception of the presentation format and the testing to be conducted on the data.

The result of this negligence is an inefficient use of resources. It results in either too much investment in information breadth and exactness, or inadequacy of information. Both can prevent the study in achieving its own underlying purposes.

9.3.1. Validity of information

Random error and systematic bias can be expected in collected dietary data. It is the responsibility of the scientist to assess the extent of these effects and their potential impact on study findings.

Random error can take place in the sampling stage of study group selection, in the reporting of usual food intake and in the estimation of nutrient levels which are consumed yearly. The first mentioned case of random error would be the accidental result, where the randomly selected population group is not representative of the reference population. Random errors can and do occur in the reporting of dietary intake, particularly in under- and over-estimation of the amounts consumed.

Systematic error (in the form of biases) can also be found in the areas of subject selection, reported intakes, and the information content of food composition tables. In the former case there are difficulties in motivating a truly representative sample to participate, and in acquiring equally valid information across age, sex, social class groups, and different income groups. For example, women are generally better reporters than men, adults than children, and individuals, from both extremely high income groups and from lower social classes, are less likely to participate in complex dietary surveys which involve either a considerable subject burden or effort.

An example of systematic bias in food composition tables is the inappropriately high levels of iron in food reported in the *USDA handbook no. 8*,[18] due to laboratory methodological problems. An overview of potential sources of error in one commonly used method of dietary assessment, the 24-hour recall, is found in Table 9.5, from the data collection stage through to the statistical analysis of the information for testing hypotheses (Fig. 9.1).

Depending on the conclusions the scientist or policy maker wishes to draw from the information base, a critical assessment of the possible

Table 9.5. Potential sources of error in the 24-hour recall method[6]

1. Question the individual about what was eaten the previous day	Memory failure Interviewer related bias
2. Question the individual about the amounts of these foods eaten	Memory failure Estimation difficulties Non-edible portions (bones, pips, etc.)
3. Code foods into machine-readable form (usually numbers)	Few codes — information compromise Reading/writing errors
4. Convert portion sizes into gram amounts	Plate waste, refuse deduction Portion size calculation from recipe
5. Enter subject identification, date, meals, foods, and amounts	Transcription errors
6. Check entered data for correctness	Oversight; difficult forms No printout of food names
7. Correct the errors	Renewed typing errors
8. Recheck the entered corrections	Oversight or elimination of this step altogether
9. Merge this information into a common database with food nutrient information and calculate out the average nutrient intake for the day	Programmes with irregular mathematical procedures Unchecked programmes
10. Group foods for comparison of frequency and amounts consumed of basic food groups between individuals	Double counting, mistakes in grouping
11. Compare intake of nutrients between case and control groups	Missing values in nutrient tables cause artificial differences
12. Test for significant differences between groups	Invalid methods selected

sources and extent of random error and systematic bias should be undertaken. This is particularly important if statements about the nutritional status of a population are being made and it should be insured that the underlying sample was representative of the total population structure. If this is found not to be the case, corrective measures are recommended such as weighting the sub-samples to a total population profile.

Measurement of error and estimation of bias are treated mathematically in Chapter 10. A close examination of the impact of bias on intake estimations can be found in a report of the National Research

Council Subcommittee on Criteria for Dietary Evaluation entitled *Nutrient adequacy, assessment, and using food consumption surveys.*[14] Through estimation of systematic bias in intake, it shows that the bias of the estimate can be great, despite relatively small systematic errors. It also shows that the magnitude of the effect of systematic bias on the estimate of the prevalence of an adequate intake, is dependent on the position of the distribution of intake in the population.

Furthermore, the probability of bias in the assessment of specific nutrient adequacy differs greatly from nutrient to nutrient. For example, the state of assessment methodology of vitamins B_{12}, C, and folate in foods is such that, at best, poor estimates of intake can be expected from most food consumption studies.

The number of foods in a dietary record has a positive impact on the error term for computed nutrient intake, as proven by the Subcommittee on Criteria for Dietary Evaluation. The effect of error of measurement variation and food composition can be computed by the following equation:[14]

$$V = I^2 \times V_c + C^2 \times V_I + V_{(c)} \times V_{(I)}$$

where: V = Estimate of variance of intake and composition
$\quad\quad V_I$ = Variance of intake measurement
$\quad\quad V_c$ = Variance of composition measurement
$\quad\quad I$ = Reported mean intake of units of food
$\quad\quad C$ = Reported mean concentration of nutrient per unit of food.

9.3.2. Variation

A number of sources of true variation must be considered in the interpretation of dietary and nutrient information. One of the most important of these is day-to-day and seasonal variation in intake behaviour of the individual. Quantification of this is discussed in Chapter 10. The size of the quotient of within- to between-person variation is an important determinant of the number of recorded days required to adequately test the hypotheses in question.

Another area of variability is in the true nutrient content of a given amount of food, between food samples. For example, the difference in vitamin C content of different species of orange or carotene content of different carrots. This issue is confounded by sampling and terminology problems, where the food, actually analysed and presented in the food composition table, may not be an appropriate comparable specimen to the product available on the market. Seasonal differences in nutrient content of specific items need also be considered, such as the vitamin D content of milk. The trace element values of foods are determined by soil characteristics. Quantification of this soil variability in food composition data, as well as variability due to sampling procedures and random variability in the food concerned is discussed in depth in Chapter 8.

9.3.3. Bioavailability

Analysts, attempting to answer the question of the consumed diet in terms of nutrient intake adequacy, require courage in their interpretation in terms of knowledge or ignorance about the bioavailability of the individual nutrient under discussion. Unfortunately our knowledge of bioavailability is limited.

Futhermore, we often base intake estimates on information of the nutrient content of a raw food, which is actually subsequently processed and prepared under unknown time and temperature conditions, and in combination with other foods. Here too, basic knowledge on nutrient losses and gains, and the availability as affected by other ingredients, is scanty. The amount of nutrient, that actually crosses the gut and becomes available, or contributes to the nutrient stores and the resources of the individual, is the next in a series of question marks.

9.3.4. Missing values

Despite the best intentions and in studies meticulously carried out, the missing value issue will raise its ugly head at various levels of information. Approaches to filling in missing gaps and minimizing the damage of missing information should be considered in the data analysis stages. If, and when this option is not taken, the effect of information gaps needs to be considered in the interpretation of results.

In dietary surveys, missing values appear as missing days or meals of intake, missing amounts of food consumed, inadequate descriptive information for useful coding at the individual level, absence of the consumed food in food composition tables, or missing values for the nutrients in question in food composition tables; and, in a broader sense, the non-participants in a representative random sample study (8.3.3, 8.3.7 and 8.5.1).

The interpreter of the data analysis should be fully aware of the extent to which analyses are based on analyses of incomplete information and the effects due to the fact that out of necessity, missing values have been treated as zeros in the analyses.

References

1. Arab, L., Schellenberg, B., and Schlierf, G., (1982). Nutrition and health—a

survey of young men and women in Heidelberg. *Ann. Nutr. Metab.* (suppl 1), **26**, 244 pp.

2. Arab, L. (1986). Coding and entry of food intakes. *Proceedings of the Eighth National Nutrient Data Bank Conference.* pp. 13–22, National Technical Information Service, Minneapolis, Springfield, VA.
3. Arab, L. (1986). Computer assisted dietary assessment. In: *Proceedings of the XIII International Congress of Nutrition* (Tailor, T. G. and Jenkins, N. K. eds) John Libbey, London.
4. Arab, L. Towards a merged European food composition database. *Proceedings of the EUROFOODS meeting, 25–28 August 1985, Norwich* (in press).
5. Arab, L. *Dietary methodology considerations for HANES III: Summary of the planning workshop for HANES III,* National Center for Health Statistics, Washington, DC (in press).
6. Arab, L., Fischer, E., Heeschen, W., Hoffmeister, H., Hötzel, D., Kohlmeier, M., Kübler, W., Rottka, H., Schlierf, G., Schmidt-Gayk, H., and Thefeld, W. (1985). Design of the nutrition and health study of elderly in Heidelberg, Michelstadt, and Berlin. *IV European Nutrition Congress, Amsterdam, May 24–27, 1983.* (Van den Berg, E. M. E., Bosman, W., and Breedveld, B. C., eds). p. 158. Voorlichtingsbureau voor de Voeding, The Hague, The Netherlands.
7. Beaton, G. H. (1986). Toward harmonization of dietary, biochemical, and clinical assessments. The meanings of nutritional status and requirements. *Nutr. Rev.* **44**, 349–58.
8. Bellin, O. and Arab, L. (1984). ESSEKAN; Ein standardisiertes 24-stunden erinnerungsprotokoll über körperliche aktivatät und nahrungsmittelaufnahme. In: *BFE, Bundesforschungsanstalt füer Ernährung.* (Engesserstrasse 20, D-7509 Karlsruhe 1, Germany.)
9. Cleveland, W. (1979). Robust locally weighted regression and smoothing scatterplots. *J. Am. Stat. Assoc.* **74**, 829.
10. Cochran, W., and Snedecor, G. (1967). *Statistical methods.* The Iowa State University Press, Ames, Iowa.
11. Eisensmith, S. P. PLOT IT: User's guide. January 1986.
12. Harris, R. (1975). *A primer of multivariate statistics.* Academic Press, New York.
13. Hoover, L. W. (ed.) (1986). *Nutrient data base directory,* (5th edition). University of Missouri, Columbia Printing Services, Columbia, Mo.
14. National Research Council Subcommittee on Criteria for Dietary Evaluation (1986). *Nutrient adequacy, assessment, and using food consumption surveys.* National Academic Press, Washington, DC.
15. Rothman, K. (1986). *Modern epidemiology.* Little, Brown, Boston/Toronto.
16. Cary, N. C. (1985). *SAS users guide: basics.* SAS Institute Inc.
17. Nie, N. H. (1970; 1975). *SPSS: Statistical package for the social sciences.* McGraw-Hill, London.
18. USDA. (1976–86). Composition of foods, raw, processed, prepared. *Agricultural Handbook no 8.1 to 8.14.* USDA, Washington, DC.

10

Validity and reproducibility

JAN BUREMA, WIJA A. VAN STAVEREN,
AND PIET A. VAN DEN BRANDT

10.1. Concepts of validation

In food consumption studies, the assessment of dietary intake may be accomplished in various ways. Therefore, there is a need to compare the performance of any two different methods of measurement. More specifically, the results of a new method of dietary assessment need to be validated against a common method that is of general acceptance. Because there is no 'gold' standard, only the *relative* validity of a new method can be assessed. Therefore, a validation study is said to assess the *relative* or *comparative* validity.

10.1.1. Sources of error and variation

In Chapter 6 the possibilities and limitations of methods assessing food consumption have been described. Clearly there is uncertainty about the quality of these methods. Chapter 3 (Fig. 3.3) has indicated that different sources of error and variation affect the quality of measurements. What are these sources of error and variation inherent in the observation?

1. Systematic defects in information: due to the discrepancy between what the investigator wants to estimate and what the technique actually estimates.
2. Systematic and random response error: due to the questionnaire's instructions, contents, and wording, the ability of the respondent, skill of the interviewer, and the research setting.
3. Biological within-person variation: referring to the true variation in the current daily food intake of a person, which is dependent on the food pattern.
4. Between-person variation: referring to the variation between people of their habitual food intake. This variation is inversely related to the homogeneity of the group regarding food pattern.

10.1.2. Measures of quality of a method

The quality of the measurements is determined by the validity and reproducibility of the method (Chapter 3.4). Validity is associated with
systematic (i.e. non-random) error; reproducibility with random error.
Table 10.1 gives the terms used to qualify measurements and their
association with these two types of error. The concept of accuracy
incorporates elements of both validity and reproducibility.

Table 10.1. Terms used to qualify measurements and their association
with two types of error*

Concept	Bias	Variability
Type of error	Non-random	Random
Used in this chapter	Validity Comparative or relative validity	Reproducibility
Synonyms	Unbiasedness Concurrent validity	Precision Reliability Repeatability Replicatability
	Accuracy*	

*The terms mentioned in this table refer to only one of the two types of error. In
addition, the term accuracy is used when referring to both types of error.

10.1.3. Purpose of the study

It is obvious that the demands on the quality of the estimates are
dependent on the purpose of the study in which the method will be used
and the kind of information required. Chapter 6 explains that in nutrition
research dietary data* may require different types of information:

1. Type 1: Mean consumption of a group of individuals.
2. Type 2: Mean and distribution of consumption in a group.
3. Type 3: The relative magnitude of the consumption of an individual
    (rank order).
4. Type 4: The absolute magnitude of the consumption of an individual.

   In examining the quality of a method, the type of information required
for the investigation to be carried out, determines which criteria should
be met for the method to give valid results.

*'Dietary data' includes nutrients and foods as well as meal pattern variables.

10.2. Guidelines on how to validate the selected method

Two ways of validating a dietary assessment method can be distinguished. The new method may be compared with another method designed to measure the same kind of dietary data. This kind of validation is dealt with in this chapter.

Alternatively, the new method may be validated against some external criterion (e.g. a biological marker). Chapter 11 gives references to some examples of this kind of validation study.

10.2.1. Design of a validation study

When comparing two methods of dietary assessment, it is essential to do measurements by either method on the same subjects. These measurements should refer to the same period and their errors should be independent.

Practical considerations, however, may limit the possibility to meet both requirements at the same time. For instance, when a single day record method is used as the reference method, it is quite conceivable that recalling on the next day, the food consumption of the previous 24 hours will result in correlated errors.

To avoid this problem, it is commonly assumed that group results on the same day of the week (say: Thursday) in successive weeks are similar. Thus, in practice the 24-hour recall method may be conducted on one Thursday and the 24-hour record method carried out on the next Thursday, or *vice versa*. In other words, although individual differences between the dietary intakes on successive Thursdays may exist, for a group these differences are assumed to cancel out making a fair comparison between the two methods possible. Since the individual differences affect the precision of the estimation of a potential bias between both methods, the demands on sample size requirements of such a design are serious.

To examine whether the second measurement is influenced by the first, a cross-over design may be applied. This means that the participants are randomly allocated to two groups. One group starts with the 24-hour recall method and the other group with the 24-hour record method. However, the demands on sample size of such a design are even more serious.

10.2.2. Estimation of bias

For the estimation of bias it is sufficient to know the differences between the paired observations, $d_i = y_i - x_i$, where:

d_i = the difference between y_i and x_i;
y_i = an observation obtained by the method to be tested;
x_i = an observation obtained by the reference method.

From the sample of n subjects, we can calculate the mean of these differences:

$$\bar{d} = \frac{1}{n}\Sigma d_i, \text{ where } i = 1, 2, \ldots, n.$$

For satisfactory validity, this mean should be as small as possible. A confidence interval for the unknown true difference between the methods may be constructed by means of the estimated variance of the differences:

$$S_d^2 = \frac{1}{n-1}\Sigma(d_i - \bar{d})^2 = \frac{1}{n-1}(\Sigma d_i^2 - (\Sigma d_i)^2/n).$$

Specifically, the lower and upper $(1 - \alpha)100$ per cent confidence limits are approximately:

$$D_{lower} = \bar{d} - w,$$
$$D_{upper} = \bar{d} + w,$$

where:

$$w = Z_{a/2}\sqrt{S_d^2/n}$$

and where, for large n, $Z_{a/2}$ may be taken as the upper $(\alpha/2)100$ per cent point of a standard normal (Gaussian) distribution. So, for a 95 per cent confidence interval (CI): $Z_{a/2} = 1.96$ and for a 90 per cent CI $Z_{a/2} = 1.645$. For values of n smaller than 30, $Z_{a/2}$ should be replaced by the corresponding $t_{a/2}$-value from a t-distribution with $n - 1$ degrees of freedom.

Example 10.1

In 22 men nitrogen (N) intake was assessed by the dietary history method (DH) and estimated from urine N-excretion/24 hours including 2 g for extra renal N losses.[12] The mean of the individual differences was 0.2 g (DH − urine excretion) with a standard error of 0.94. Since the standard error is equal to the standard deviation/$\sqrt{n}$, and $t_{a/2} = 2.08$ for $\alpha = 0.05$ and $n - 1 = 21$, the confidence limits may be calculated as:

$$0.2 - 2.08 \times 0.94 = -1.8 \text{ g, and}$$
$$0.2 + 2.08 \times 0.94 = 2.2 \text{ g.}$$

These data do not indicate that the difference between the N-intake from the dietary history and the N-excretion was different from zero. We conclude that these data do not support evidence for the presence of a bias and, thus, that the dietary history method is relatively valid as far as the assessment of protein is concerned (N × 6.25). (NB: if $Z_{a/2} = 1.96$ is used rather than $t_{a/2}$, the confidence limits become -1.6 and 2.0, respectively.)

10.2.3. Non-constant bias

If the purpose of the investigation is to assess the *distribution* of the intake of a nutrient (type 2 information) or to obtain estimates of individual habitual intakes (type 4 information), one should consider the possibility of non-constant bias. This means that the degree of over- or under-estimation is dependent on whether the intake is low or high.

An example of non-constant bias is the so-called flat slope syndrome: those who eat more under-estimate their intake and those who are small eaters tend to over-estimate their intake. A proper evaluation of this phenomenon, however, involves serious statistical intricacies which are rarely appreciated in the literature.

Although it is common to calculate a regression line of *y* on *x* in this situation, this may lead to misinterpretation due to regression towards the mean.

To exclude the possibility of a non-constant, level dependent bias, it is recommended that the association between the differences d_i and the sums, $t_i = y_i + x_i$, should be tested. This may be done either by testing whether the regression coefficient of *d* on *t* is zero ($\beta_{dt} = 0$), or by testing whether the correlation coefficient between the difference and the sum is zero ($\rho_{dt} = 0$). If this hypothesis is rejected, the assumption of a *constant* bias is invalid. Consequently, any statement about the presence or absence of a bias in the second method, when compared with the first method, is only valid for a specific range of intake. Thus, in case of non-constant bias, a statement on bias which does not specify its range of application would be meaningless.

10.2.4. Evaluation of the validity of a method

The validity of a method of dietary assessment depends on the purpose of the study. When the aim is to assess the association between a dietary component and some other variable, such as serum cholesterol or incidence of cardiovascular disease or cancer, a correct *ranking* of subjects as to their dietary intake is of importance (cf. 10.1.3 type 3 information). To achieve this, it is not a prerequisite for a method to be free of bias. This situation is dealt with in a subsequent paragraph (10.2.6).

When the difference between two group means is to be tested, the dietary intake of both groups being measured by the same method, a constant bias may do no harm to the resulting conclusion. However, a non-constant bias may affect the power of the test and thus produce a false negative result.

In other cases, a constant bias invalidates the results of the study, for example when estimation of the exact level of mean intake in a group is the aim of the study (type 1 information). This is also true when the distribution (standard deviation, percentiles) of dietary intake in a group is the object of the study (type 2 information), or when the absolute amounts of dietary intake of an individual should be estimated (type 4 information).

10.2.5. Sample size in a validation study

Calculation of the required number of subjects (observations) N, needed for a specific precision in the estimation of the bias, presumes some knowledge about the variance of differences d_i, σ_d^2.

In 10.2.2, this variance was estimated from the data as S_d^2. However, sample size should be decided before the beginning of the study. From prior knowledge an estimation of the within-person coefficients of variation of each of the methods being compared, CV_A and CV_B, may be available. These may be used to assess an estimation of the variance of the differences d_i:

$$\sigma_d^2 = (CV_A^2 + CV_B^2) \times (\text{mean level of dietary intake})^2.$$

After deciding on the required precision of the estimation of the bias by choosing the width, $2w$, of its confidence interval, the required number of observations may be calculated from:

$$n = (Z_{a/2})^2 \, (\sigma_d^2 / w^2).$$

When w is expressed as a fraction of the mean dietary intake, say:

$$w = f \times (\text{mean intake})$$

then:

$$n = (Z_{a/2})^2 \, \frac{CV_A^2 + CV_B^2}{f^2} .$$

Alternatively, f and CV may all be expressed as a percentage, rather than a fraction.

Example 10.2.

In 123 young adult women, protein intake was assessed by Method A: 14 monthly repeated 24-hour recalls and Method B: from N-excretion (N × 6.25) in 14 collections of 24-hour urine, including 2 g (N × 6.25) for extra renal N losses.[13]

	Mean intake $(\bar{x})$	Within-person variation (s)	CV^2 $(s/\bar{x})^2$
Method A	68.1	8.8	0.017
Method B	65.5	13.0	0.039

For assessment of the required sample size of a similar study on the relative validity of method A, an estimate of σ_d^2 may be derived from these data:

$$\hat{\sigma}_d^2 = (0.017 + 0.039) \times (65.5)^2.$$

If the required precision (w) is 10 per cent of the mean intake, where w is the half width of a 95 per cent confidence interval and thus $Z_{\alpha/2} = 1.96$, then the minimum sample size is:

$$n = (1.96)^2 \frac{0.017 + 0.039}{(0.10)^2} = 3.84 \times 5.6 = 22.$$

10.2.6. When ranking of subjects is the objective

When nutrition is investigated in the context of the etiology of a disease, associations may be calculated between dietary intake (energy or nutrients) and other, non-dietary variables. If these variables have a continuous distribution, for example, blood pressure, body weight, serum cholesterol, the results of the study may be expressed as regression coefficients or as correlation coefficients, for example (Pearson's) product-moment correlation coefficients or (Spearman's) rank order correlation coefficients.

In order to obtain valid conclusions from such a study, it is not neces-sary for the dietary assessment method to be free of bias. A method that has a constant bias may produce the same associations with external variables as a bias-free method would do.

So, when only correct ranking of subjects as to their dietary intake is the objective (type 3 information), how should a new method be validated against a reference method?

Though absence of bias is no longer a prerequisite, *linearity* of the relationship between the values of both methods is a sufficient condition for the product-moment correlation coefficient to be unchanged. The weaker condition of a *monotonous* relationship is sufficient to leave the rank order correlation coefficient unchanged.

Whether each of these conditions holds for the new method under consideration, may be evaluated by calculating the correspondent correlation coefficient between paired measurements, which should be close to one. However, violation of the above assumption is not the only reason for the correlation coefficient to be smaller than one. An imperfect association may also be caused by a poor reproducibility of the dietary assessment.

When subjects are classified into categories of dietary intake, either with fixed limits or based on quantiles of the distribution (tertiles, quintiles, etc.), another measure of agreement between two methods is Cohen's kappa. This is the proportion of classifications in the same category according to either method, corrected for chance.[6]

Sample size considerations such as in the preceding paragraph do not carry over to the present situation. It seems wise practice to take at least 50 subjects. In addition, the between-person variation should be similar to the variation in the population to be investigated.

10.3. Reproducibility

10.3.1. The need for knowledge of variability

The investigator who is to design a study on dietary data, needs some information about variability in order to determine the sample size required to attain a specific degree of precision. When the objective of the study is to estimate the individual mean value for a subject, the within-person variation is the relevant piece of information. This may be expressed as a standard deviation, S_{within}, or as coefficient of variation:

$$CV_{within} = S_{within}/(\text{mean level of intake}).$$

When estimation of a group mean is the issue, the between-subject variation is also needed. Generally the estimated total variance will be available. This is the sum of intra-individual and inter-individual variance:

$$S^2_{total} = S^2_{within} + S^2_{between}.$$

When assessment of the association with an external variate is the ultimate goal, the degree of attenuation (inflation, dilution, bias to null) of such an estimate is determined by the ratio of within- and between-person variability.[2,8,11]

Example 10.3.

Van Staveren *et al.*[14] estimated the fatty acid composition of sub-cutaneous adipose tissue and diet in 59 young adult women. Food consumption was estimated by the mean of nineteen 24-hour recalls administered over a period of 2.5 years. Highly significant correlations were found between linoleic acid content of the diet and the fat tissue ($r = 0.70$).

When using one 24-hour recall instead of the average of 19 recalls, the correlation coefficient was substantially decreased (approximately 0.28).

The ratio of within- and between-person variance in linoleic acid was 1.8 in this study.

This demonstrates the weakening effect (attenuation) of the large day-to-day variation in within-person intake on the correlation coefficient.

10.3.2. Time frame

For methods designed to assess an individual's 24-hour dietary intake, day-to-day variability in intake is a source of variation that contributes to the within-person variance.

On the other hand, a dietary history relating to a period of 1, 2, or 3 months is not sensitive for short-term fluctuations. It may, however, be affected by seasonal variations.

Thus, when within-person variability of dietary assessment is studied, the results should be related explicitly to the time frame of that particular dietary method.

10.3.3. Design of a reproducibility study

Reproducibility refers to variability of a measurement on the *same* subject, under the *same* condition. This latter phrase deserves further explanation. It would be meaningless, for example, to ask a person to record his food intake twice on the *same day*.

Repeated measurements on the same subject, therefore, will necessarily relate to different days, or periods. Thus a source of variation other than those due to the technique itself, is inevitably included in the within-person variation.

Consequently, to assess reproducibility, for each subject, two (or more) measurements are needed relating to periods in time that, although different, are as similar as possible.

10.3.4. Estimation of reproducibility

As a measure of reproducibility of a single measurement, the intra-individual variance of the dietary assessment is recommended:

$$S^2_{\text{within}}.$$

Alternatively, the standard deviation, $S_{\text{within}} = (S^2_{\text{within}})^{1/2}$, may be preferred, or better still the coefficient of variation,

$$CV_{\text{within}} = S_{\text{within}}/\text{mean}.$$

In the case of uncorrelated observations per person, the variance of the differences between pairs of observations is equal to twice the intra-individual variance. Thus, the latter may be estimated as:

$$S^2_{\text{within}} = \frac{1}{2(n-1)} \Sigma(d_i - \bar{d})^2$$

where d_i is the individual difference, and the summation is over n subjects.

The use of $\bar{d}$, the mean difference in the group, as an indicator of 'reproducibility on the group level' should be strongly discouraged. It is, in fact, either an estimate of some unintended time effect, or just a particular realization of a random variable with mean zero and variance equal to twice the variance of the estimate of a group mean. As such, it has no relevance. For studies aiming at assessment of group means (type 1 information), an estimate of the total variance would be a meaningful measure of the reproducibility of estimating group means.

In the case of three or more observations per subject, the residual error variance may be established from an analysis of variance model. For one proper model to estimate the coefficient of variation, see van Staveren.[14]

10.4. Validity and reproducibility studies in the literature

In the last decade several review articles have been published on the possibilities and limitations of methods assessing food consumption.[1-5, 7, 9, 10] However, great care must be taken in drawing general conclusions regarding the validity and reproducibility of these methods. The reason is that most studies on validating methods have been conducted with different purposes, in different research settings, and with different population groups. The validity and reproducibility of methods assessing food consumption is affected by these factors. Another reason to be careful when drawing general conclusions, is that authors publishing validity studies have not always made clear the type of information required to use these methods for the purpose of their research.

Futhermore the research design and the statistics applied to examine validity and reproducibility were not always appropriate.

The tabulated scheme showing which method may be used for the various purposes (Chapter 6) is based on the experience of the authors and on literature research. As already mentioned, the validity and reproducibility of methods to assess food consumption depend on many factors. Almost always in nutrition research these methods should be adapted for specific research purposes, research setting, population groups with specific disabilities and food habits.

Before applying a method in these various research designs under different circumstances, it should always be tested first.

This chapter has explained how the methods to collect different types of information might be tested for relative validity and reproducibility. Chapter 11 will review problems of validation studies in practice.

References

1. Bazarre, T. L. and Myers, M. P. (1979). The collection of food intake data in cancer epidemiology studies. *Nutr. Cancer* **4**, 22–45.
2. Beaton, G. H., Milner, J., Corey, P., *et al.* (1979). Sources of variance in 24-hour dietary recall data: implications for nutrition study design and interpretation. *Am. J. Clin. Nutr.* **32**, 2546–59.
3. Bingham, S. (1983). Premise and methods. In: *Surveillance of the dietary habits of the population with regard to cardiovascular disease.* (De Backer, G., Tunstall Pedoe, H., and Ducimetière, P., eds). pp 21–42. EURO-NUT report 2. Wageningen.
4. Block, G. (1982). A review of validations of dietary assessment methods. *Am. J. Epidemiol.* **115**. 492–505.
5. Burk, M. C. and Pao, E. M. (1976). Methodology for large scale surveys of household and individual diets. *Home Economic Report no. 40.* USDA, Washington.
6. Fleiss, J. L. (1973). *Statistical methods for rates and proportions.* pp. 143–55. Wiley & Sons, New York.
7. Krantzler, N. J., Muller, J., Comstock, E. M. *et al.* (1982). Methods of food intake assessment—an annotated bibliography. *J. Nutr. Ed.* **14**, 108–19.
8. Liu, K., Stamler, J., Dyer, A., McKeever, J., and McKeever, P. (1978). Statistical methods to assess and minimize the role of intra-individual variability in obscuring the relationship between dietary lipids and serum cholesterol. *J. Chron. Dis.* **31**, 399–418.
9. Marr, J. W. (1971). Individual dietary surveys: purposes and methods. *Wld Rev. Nutr. Diet.* **13**, 105–64.
10. Pekkarinen, M. (1970). Methodology in the collection of food consumption data. *Wld Rev. Nutr. Diet.* **12**, 277–94.
11. Sempos, C., Johnson, M. E. W., Smith, E. L. and Gillican, C. (1985). Effects of intra-individual variation in repeated dietary records. *Am. J. Epidemiol.* **121**, 120–30.
12. Staveren, W. A. van, de Boer, J. O., and Burema, J. (1985). Validity and reproducibility of a dietary history method estimating the usual food intake during one month. *Am. J. Clin. Nutr.* **42**, 554–9.
13. Staveren, W. A. van. (1985). *Dietary intake methods: their validity and reproducibility.* PhD thesis. Wageningen, The Netherlands.
14. Staveren, W. A. van, Deurenberg, P., Katan, M. B. *et al.* (1986). Validity of the fatty acid composition of subcutaneous fat tissue microbiopsies as an estimate of the long-term average fatty acid composition of the diet of individuals. *Am. J. Epidemiol.* **123**, 455–63.

11

Validation problems

JEAN H. HANKIN

Introduction

As discussed in Chapter 10, the validity of a dietary method is its ability to measure the intakes of foods or nutrients with accuracy (3.4). Validation of a dietary recall or history is a problem because there is no absolute standard for estimating the true usual intakes of free-living persons.[1, 15, 16] Consequently, investigators have selected various criteria as standards for validating the selected dietary method for a particular study.

At the outset, it should be noted that demonstrations of reproducibility are not substitutes for tests of validity. Reproducibility or reliability is a measure of the repeatability of a method administered on two occasions to the same individuals (3.4.3). Although data from two surveys may agree, this could be due to the repetition of the same error in the method on the two occasions. It follows that a dietary method may be evaluated as 'unreliable' but, at the same time, be a questionable validity.

This chapter will concentrate on the validation of a dietary recall or history and will review some of the problems of validation, look at two examples of methods used in validity studies, and make recommendations for future research in this area.

11.1. Four major problems in validation

There are four major problem areas to discuss, the first being the variability in the accuracy of recall. The literature includes a number of papers in which individuals were unknowingly observed during a meal or a 24-hour period.[2-4, 9, 11]

Quantities of foods were first measured and subjects were subsequently questioned about foods and the amounts consumed. There was variability in the accuracy of recalls among the various populations. A warning is needed to interpret these studies with caution. Even though agreement might be satisfactory, the validation of a particular meal or single day's intake provides no indication of the validity of a person's usual diet during a relatively long time period. Furthermore, many of these studies were conducted in schools or institutions where the meals may differ considerably from the usual eating patterns elsewhere.

A second problem relates to the memory error which is likely to occur among persons asked to recall their past diet. In case–control studies investigators wish to obtain data on diet before diagnosis or onset of symptoms in the cases and within a comparable time period in the controls. Perfect recall is not expected. Although memory errors may occur, these errors are likely to affect responses concerning past diet among the cases and controls. Because cases may alter their diets after diagnosis and counselling, it is particularly important to emphasize the desired time period for the recall.

In a cohort study in which healthy subjects are to be followed for a period of time to assess disease incidence or mortality, a more recent dietary history, such as the previous month, may be used. In this situation, it would be expected that a dietary recall would be less of a problem than in case–control studies.

The third problem relates to the dietary analysis of the food intakes. For large population studies, nutritionists need to select appropriate food composition tables for computing the nutrient intakes. Various data sets have been published by governmental units of several countries and a number of private scientific groups (Table 8.2). In general, the data are from various sources and the composition of a particular item is not fixed or consistent. It may differ in various geographic areas and during seasons of the year (8.2.2). To increase the validity of the dietary intakes, it would be desirable to develop recipes which used various local food combinations. These food mixes and any other important local or regional foods would be sent for laboratory analysis. Such values should then be added to the food composition data bank. Although food composition errors would affect the validity of the computed dietary intakes, they may not necessarily affect the comparisons of cases and controls.

A fourth major problem is the difference in validating the diets of a few subjects in a metabolic or laboratory study and the diets of a large population in an epidemiological study. In the first situation, precise data on the intakes of particular nutrients, such as micrograms of retinol or milligrams of ascorbic acid, are looked for. In the second study, the dietary data may be used to classify individuals on a continuum from low to high intakes of selected foods or nutrients or to classify subjects into broad categories of increasing intake (type 3 information). If the dietary method and the standard criteria classify the subjects in a relatively similar way, this could be interpreted as high validity of the method. This classification may be sufficient, if the purpose is to confirm or test an association between diet and disease. However, greater precision may be needed if valid recommendations were to be made to the public about intake levels below, or above which a risk is increased.

11.2. Reported validation methods

11.2.1. Dietary

Most investigators develop or select dietary history methods believed to yield reasonably accurate food consumption data for a study. These methods have been validated among representative samples of the study population by comparison with weighed, measured, or estimated intakes,[5, 7, 8] during a week or longer time period. Although some persons may modify their eating patterns to simplify their record-keeping, this method does provide more accurate and precise intake data than a dietary history. Relative agreement of the two methods would indicate acceptable validity.

As already suggested, there is always a question about the ability of individuals to recall the foods they consumed several months, or even years ago. Yet, van Leeuwen *et al.*[8] had considerable success in testing the validity of a dietary history method designed to estimate dietary intakes recorded 4 years previously. In 1981, 79 men and women were interviewed about their food intakes in 1977. The results were compared with those obtained in the same group by 7-day records in 1977. Differences in the mean intakes of energy and nutrients were generally less than 10 per cent. Correlations of the nutrient intakes ranged from 0.38 for animal protein to 0.68 for energy, total and saturated fat, and polysaccharides. Also, when the population was divided by tertiles of intake of various nutrients, the proportions in the same thirds were generally between 47 and 70 per cent.

Another approach has been reported by Jain *et al.*,[7] who compared a dietary history method with food records among 16 husband–wife pairs. Unknown to the husbands, the wives kept measured records of the men's diets for a period of 30 days. Using the dietary history method, Jain then interviewed the men for a recall of their food intakes during the same period of time. Although mean nutrient intakes were somewhat higher for the histories than the records, the estimated values from both methods were positively correlated.

Willett and his group[14] evaluated the validity of a 61-item semi-quantitative food frequency questionnaire used in a large prospective study among 173 nurses. The questionnaire was used twice at an interval of a year and four 1-week diet records were collected within that period. They found that the mean nutrient intakes from the records correlated more strongly with the questionnaires after adjusting for total energy intake. They also reported good agreement between the methods in placing subjects in the same high or low fifths of the distribution of energy-adjusted intakes of several nutrients.

Hankin and co-workers,[6] have tested the validity of their dietary history method. A random sample of approximately 300 men and women recorded their food intakes during a 1-week period at 3-month intervals, four times a year. The subjects were given a small notebook for recording food items consumed and a book with photographs of 47 frequently consumed foods, showing three serving sizes, labelled A, B, and C (Fig. 7.2). After each meal, the subject checked the book for items eaten and recorded the number of A, B, and C servings consumed. Nothing was measured. Then, 6 months after the fourth record set, an interviewer visited the subject and obtained a history of the usual frequencies of intake and estimated amounts of the same 47 items consumed between the first to the fourth record weeks. This procedure simulates typical case-control studies in which people are often interviewed 6 or more months after diagnosis of disease. By using the same format for the records and histories and the same quantifying methods, the investigators would be able to measure the validity of the recall itself against the mean intakes of the four weekly food records.

11.2.2. Biological

It would be ideal to identify particular biological or biochemical markers which would validate or perhaps estimate long-range individual nutrient intakes. However, there are at least two major problems in this area. First, levels of some nutrients in plasma, serum, or urine are regulated more by physiological mechanisms than by diet. Included in this group of nutrients are cholesterol, vitamin A, and calcium. Second, the levels of nutrients sensitive to dietary intakes, such as carotene and ascorbic acid, tend to reflect recent intakes rather than past usual consumption. This is a problem similar to the use of recent food records to validate dietary histories. However, if various types of measurement demonstrate relative agreement, this would suggest that these validation methods may be appropriate for assessing past, as well as recent intakes.[1]

The use of nutrient levels in urine, blood, and faecal material to estimate dietary intakes is not a new procedure. For some time, investigators have analysed these materials for nitrogen, sodium, and various minerals and vitamins in metabolic studies. However, their use as biochemical markers to validate dietary histories has not been reported until recently and a few examples are included in this chapter.

Van Staveren *et al.*[12] used 24-hour urinary nitrogen excretions to validate 1-month dietary histories obtained from 44 adults. Agreement between nitrogen excretion and intakes among the group was 0.0 g with

95 per cent confidence limits of ± 1.1 g. However, at the individual level there was considerable variation between intakes and excretions of nitrogen. Of course, as the authors pointed out, there cannot be a generalization about the validity of other nutrients from data on a single dietary component.

In another study, Willett *et al.*[14] assessed the validity of their semi-quantitative dietary history by comparing the carotene and tocopherol intakes with the plasma levels of these nutrients in 59 adults. After adjusting for energy intakes and plasma lipids, they found significant correlations for both parameters.

Recent research suggests that some body tissues may be appropriate for validating the past intakes of particular nutrients. For example, van Staveren *et al.*[13] demonstrated a highly significant association between dietary fat intakes and the fatty acid composition of subcutaneous fat tissues. She collected nineteen 24-hour recalls from 59 women during a 2.5-year period. Then, 3 months after the completion of the dietary survey, adipose tissue samples from the buttocks of these women were collected. Correlations of 0.70 were found between the linoleic acid contents of the diet and the fat tissues and of 0.62 between the ratio of linoleic acid to saturated fatty acids of the diet and fatty tissues. It should be noted that these associations would be valid only for adults whose body weights were fairly constant during recent years.

11.3. Recommendations for further research

Further research is needed to identify additional biological markers or indicators that could be used to validate past dietary intakes. For example, other body tissues, including hair and nails, may be appropriate indicators of protein and mineral status. Similarly, there may be other indicators, such as circulating enzyme concentrations for particular minerals and vitamins and faecal metabolites for fat and fibre components, that would provide valid indicators of long-term intakes. However, the use of biological markers does introduce new dimensions to the validation problems: absorption and metabolism. There might be need to consider other factors in the equation, such as nutrient interactions in absorption, individual variation in metabolic efficiency, concurrent diseases, and weight changes.

It is likely that dietary histories, or records, and plasma samples were collected in several cohort studies conducted among large populations beginning in the 1950s. If those plasma samples were frozen and stored, they might be used for the validation of dietary histories conducted among the same subjects. Biological markers of past intake are not likely to replace estimates of dietary intake, as public health recommendations are likely to be made in terms of dietary intakes. Still, the markers could be used to test associations and to validate dietary methods.

Finally, as suggested earlier, the concept of dietary validation might well be modified. It is highly improbable that we will ever achieve precise agreement between a dietary history and standard dietary or biochemical criteria. However, it is conceivable that relative agreement between these two parameters could be achieved. If both methods place subjects in the same rank order of intake or in similar high- and low-intake categories, this would provide valid data for examining the associations between diet and disease in population studies.

References

1. Block, G. (1982). A review of validations of dietary assessment methods. *Am. J. Epidemiol.* **115**, 492–505.
2. Campbell, V. A. and Dodds, M. I. (1967). Collecting dietary information from groups of older people. *J. Am. Diet Assoc.* **51**, 29–33.
3. Emmons, L. and Hayes, M. (1973). Accuracy of 24-hour recalls of young children. *J. Am. Diet Assoc.* **62**, 409–15.
4. Greger, J. L. and Etnyre, G. (1978). Validity of 24-hour dietary recalls by adolescent females. *Am. J. Pub. Hlth.* **68**, 70–2.
5. Hankin, J. H., Rhoads, G. G. and Glober G. A. (1975). A dietary method for an epidemiologic study of gastrointestinal cancer. *Am. J. Clin. Nutr.* **28**, 1055–61.
6. Hankin, J. H. A diet history method for research, clinical and community use. *J. Am. Diet Assoc.* (in press).
7. Jain, M., Howe, G. R. and Johnson, K. C. (1980). Evaluation of a diet history questionnaire for epidemiologic studies. *Am. J. Epidemiol.* **111**, 212–19.
8. Leeuwen, F. E. van, Vet, H. C. W. de, *et al.* (1983). An assessment of the relative validity of retrospective interviewing for measuring dietary intake. *Am. J. Epidemiol.* **118**, 752–8.
9. Linusson, E. E. I., Sanjur, D. and Erickson, E. C. (1974). Validating the 24-hour recall method as a dietary survey tool. *Arch. Latinoam. Nutr.* **24**, 277–94.
10. Madden, J. P., Goodman, S. J. and Guthrie, H. A. (1976). Validity of the 24-hour recall. *J. Am. Diet Assoc.* **68**, 143–7.
11. Meredith, A., Matthews, A., Zickefoose, M. *et al.* (1951). How well do school children recall what they have eaten. *J. Am. Diet Assoc.* **27**, 749.
12. Staveren, W. A. van, Boer, J. O. de, and Burema, J. (1985). Validity and reproducibility of a dietary history method estimating the usual food intake during one month. *Am. J. Clin. Nutr.* **42**, 554–9.
13. Staveren, W. A. van, Deurenberg, P., Katan, M. B. *et al.* (1986). Validity of the fatty acid composition of subcutaneous fat tissue microbiopsies as an

estimate of the long-term average fatty acid composition of the diet of separate individuals. *Am. J. Epidemiol.* **123**, 455–63.

14. Willett, W. E. C., Stampfer, M. J., Underwood, B. A. *et al.* (1983). Validation of a dietary questionnaire with plasma carotenoid and -tocopherol levels. *Am. J. Clin. Nutr.* **38**, 631–9.

15. Willett, W. C., Sampson, L., Stampfer, H. J. *et al.* (1985). Reproducibility and validity of a semi-quantitative food frequency questionnaire. *Am. J. Epidemiol.* **122**, 51–65.

16. Young, C. M. (1981). Dietary methodology. In: *Assessing changing food consumption patterns.* pp. 89–118. National Academy of Sciences, Washington.

Acknowledgements

Appreciation is extended to Dr. Loic Le Marchand, Epidemiology Program, Cancer Research Center, University of Hawaii, and Ms. Carol Boushey, Nutritionist, School of Public Health, University of Hawaii, for review of this manuscript.

12

Obtaining food consumption data in special circumstances: additional considerations

ELIZABETH CAMPBELL ASSELBERGS AND
JEAN HENDERSON SABRY

Introduction

During the course of surveys, special circumstances can arise which demand innovative approaches to data collection. Common sense, practical solutions are required which make least demands on field-workers and subjects and on the time and funds available. This chapter suggests approaches that take into account the problems associated with surveys of people living in remote areas, of people with physical disabilities, and of those on special dietary regimens. The last section deals with problems specific to food consumption surveys in developing countries.

Population groups with particular characteristics may be randomly selected during the normal sampling procedure for a survey, or purposely selected as for a research study on a particular food, health, or other problem. In the latter case, the limitations of the study population must be kept in mind. Obvious problems must be avoided. Paraplegics, for example, should not be expected to visit clinics, nor should those who cannot write be asked to keep records. Efforts are needed so that the co-operation of the disabled is actually made easier.

In large surveys, the statistical importance of including particular groups should be weighed against the extra demands they would create. To allow them to participate, additional costs in time, personnel, and even resources would be needed to adapt the basic survey design. For example, the number of totally deaf people likely to be selected in a population-wide survey may not warrant the special preparation of fully detailed self-explanatory questionnaire forms. However, in the developing world where blindness frequently occurs, it may be advisable to design the survey so that the blind subjects can participate fully.

Statistical sampling techniques can be used to include, exclude, or over-sample people with particular characteristics, if the prevalence or location of that characteristic among the population is already known. Individuals with a particular characteristic can be excluded from the original sampling frame or they can be substituted for, at the time of initial contact, according to some pre-arranged statistical procedure. It is important that provision for such substitution is included as part of the sample selection procedure.

12.1. Areas or settlements which are remote or have difficult access

Food consumption surveys in remote areas can be particularly important for two reasons. Often the diet available to the local inhabitants is monotonously restricted. In addition, health care facilities and other services are limited or even non-existent. Survey data can be used to document the particular situation so that the programmes and services needed are introduced, monitored and evaluated.

The response rate to surveys in areas which are remote or have difficult access can be rewardingly high. People living in these areas often welcome the attention the survey gives and their involvement in it. It is particularly appreciated if they are well informed of its purpose and the survey is introduced in a way that overcomes any suspicions they may have about it.

12.1.1. Data collection techniques

The main deterrents to surveying remote areas are the costs and time involved in fielding survey teams. Postal and telephone services can offer inexpensive alternatives to face-to-face interviewing.

By postal service

Surveying by mail is viable among literate populations where the postal service is frequent and reliable. In general, subjects need to be selected in advance with correct addresses readily available. Provision should be made for pre-paid return postage. Survey questionnaires must be carefully designed to be self-explanatory and easy to complete. Short food frequency questionnaires are likely to elicit better co-operation than either 24-hour recalls or questionnaires on foods actually consumed. Householders in remote areas cannot be expected to have precise weighing scales or be willing to devote time and effort to measuring and recording details about food consumption unless encouragement, support, or even incentives are available. Useful support can be provided relatively inexpensively through locally broadcast television or radio 'spots', or through a local community worker who receives special training to promote and assist in the survey. If the population is illiterate, a local teacher, nurse, or community worker could actually be trained to conduct the survey. The quality of data may suffer, however, if the local person is not sufficiently well trained to use the questionnaire properly.

By telephone

Where a telephone service is widely available, this technology holds promise for a relatively economical survey. Costs of telephone surveys may be higher than with mailed surveys, especially if long-distance calls are required, but two-way conversation increases the rapport between participant and interviewer, and thus is likely to improve the quality of the data. Short, simple-to-answer questionnaires are easiest to conduct by telephone (7.2.3).

By survey team

The time and costs involved in sending survey teams to remote areas will be a major consideration of any such survey. Depending on the size and number of remote areas to be surveyed, it may be advantageous to set up selected survey teams to work independently of the time scheduling of other teams. It is important that all such survey teams receive the same training and supervision so that data quality is comparable. The team should consist of physically fit, compatible individuals who can stay in remote areas for days or even weeks at a time. In addition to sufficient survey resources, including equipment and forms, sleeping, cooking, and even camping facilities may need to be provided. If teams are required to walk in to remote areas, their equipment must be easy to carry. Transport, by dirt roads and over rough terrain may require four-wheel drive vehicles. If the season dictates whether roads are passable or not, it may also dictate the timing of the survey. Boats or canoes may be needed for certain areas and even air and sea planes might be used where there are no roads and distances are great. The distance between study areas and the type of transport chosen will determine the work schedules, the number of teams, and the speed with which the data can be collected. The schedule of survey teams working in isolated places needs to provide adequate leisure time and planned recreation that will help to maintain morale among team members. In remote areas, local people should be used to inform their community, in advance, of the survey and its purpose. They should also welcome the team and introduce them to the area making them aware of local customs and courtesies (14.4.3). These local survey aides can also be trained by the survey team to act as their interpreters of local languages or dialects.

Sampling

Special sampling techniques and procedures can be used to limit the geographic scatter of the sample selected from remote areas. Cluster sampling, for example, can reduce the number of such locations selected without affecting the representativeness of the sample.[2,3] This can substantially reduce the logistical demands and operating costs of the survey.

12.2. Population groups or individuals with disabilities which influence their ability to report on food consumption

Disabilities affecting sight, hearing, speech, memory, or the ability to write are particular challenges to the collection of data from affected individuals. If only one faculty is disabled, a survey method which relies on other faculties will provide the solution needed. When the survey involves the young or the aged, help will be needed from persons who eat with, or prepare the subject's food. If all the subjects in a study are disabled, more effort is needed to encourage their co-operation than when they are only occasional respondents in a population-wide survey.

12.2.1. The blind

If blind persons selected for a study are Braille literate, essential instructions, questionnaires and any other written information should be prepared in Braille. Even if data are collected by observation or interview, Braille readers will be more prepared to cooperate if their reading ability is acknowledged and used. Alternatively, tape recorders, radios, and telephones offer opportunities for communicating with the blind. Any survey technique that relies on observation of interview is appropriate. These techniques are discussed in 7.2. Techniques based on written instructions or records, however, need to be adapted for use with blind persons. Weighing or measuring food may be difficult for the blind, but some may find three-dimensional portion-size models can help them report amounts of food eaten (7.1). Otherwise, surveys should be undertaken in the individual's home where amounts of food eaten can be measured by a member of the survey team or the household. Although there are relatively higher percentages of blind people among populations in developing countries, few of them are able to read Braille. Radios and loudspeakers, which are effective means of informing the illiterate, are equally valuable for the blind. Few surveys in the developing world rely on the written word, but pictures and posters are often used. Some effort could be made to prepare cutouts or other forms so that the blind are also encouraged to participate.

12.2.2. The deaf

Carefully prepared, self-explanatory written instructions and question-naires are required when the deaf are subjects of a study. Face-to-face interviews can be made, but these are usually more difficult and time-consuming than if a respondent can hear. Interviews can be helped by using printed instructions, questionnaires, and probing techniques, or an interpreter of sign language, if this is appropriate. Replica models or pictures can help with the identification of foods and the quantity consumed (7.1.3). Obviously, telephone interviews and radio and tape supported instructions are not appropriate for the deaf. If speech is impaired, provision can be made for written responses.

12.2.3. The young

While children over 8 years of age can present valid reports of foods consumed in the previous 24 hours, particularly if careful probing is used, foods eaten by children under 8 years is best reported by the person responsible for their meals.[1] Children between 4–8 years should be interviewed along with their guardian to report foods eaten away from home. If the child goes to a day care centre or plays in the homes of friends or relatives, it may be necessary to talk with several people in order to obtain the complete information needed.

12.2.4. The elderly

Since memory fades with age, surveying older persons requires particular care. Patience and frequent probing are required. After the individual has reported all that is easily remembered, a checklist of common foods can be used to encourage complete recall. The problem of memory can be reduced if an observer record (3.2.5; 6.3) is the method of survey.

12.2.5. The physically disabled

Information about food consumption can be tape-recorded by indivi-duals who are unable to write. While the cost of recording equipment and the transcription of the tape to text are important considerations, record-ings may considerably reduce the amount of interviewer time required in surveys of the physically disabled.

12.2.6. Illiterate people

The inclusion of illiterate people in a survey makes it impractical to use either printed information or instructions, or methods which require subjects to record their own food consumption. Interviews, either face-to-face or by telephone, and techniques which rely on the observed record (6.3), are appropriate in these circumstances.

12.3. Problems of surveying groups suffering from a specific disease or groups consuming a diet modified from the normal

Many food consumption studies are undertaken specifically to investigate the relationship between diet and a particular disease. The method chosen, therefore, must allow for the validity and precision required in such research. Individuals must be fully informed of the purpose of the investigation and advised to report on their actual food consumption. Otherwise, they may consider the study a check on their compliance to a prescribed diet and report on what has been prescribed rather than on what is actually eaten. If dietary histories or food frequencies are wanted, it may be particularly difficult for respondents to differentiate between past eating practices and those of the present. The interviewer must provide appropriate help so that memories of past practices are not influenced by the present regimen.

Diets reduced in sugar, sodium, fat, protein, or gluten, for example, are particularly important in certain disease states. If specially formulated foods, or foods of modified composition, are part of the diet, they must be carefully recorded. Details from packages of commercially prepared products should be recorded and nutrient composition obtained from manufacturers. Food composition tables may need to be expanded to include the special foods and formulations reported during studies of individuals with particular diseases (8.3.6). The same approach is needed when recording the consumption of mineral, vitamin, and other dietary supplements. The composition values of special foods and of supplements must be recorded not only in surveys of persons on modified diets, but for all participants in population surveys. Brand names of vitamin and mineral supplements, their frequency and unit of consumption need to be recorded, if total nutrient consumption is to be calculated. In a clinic, the presentation of labels from popular commercial brands, or photographs of labels or packages, can help respondents to recall the brand of the supplement used. In home interviews, the containers of vitamin, mineral, or other dietary supplements should be examined by the interviewer, to identify correctly the brand name, as proposed in section 7.2.3. Composition data should be obtained from manufacturers. Nutrient composition of these supplements should be entered into the computer and coded in a manner similar to other food compositions.

12.4. Problems specific to developing countries

Because of the nature of food problems in developing countries, food consumption surveys can be particularly valuable in helping to document the type, severity, location, and causes of malnutrition and deprivation among these populations. While such surveys are known to be expensive undertakings, they can provide valuable data for policy making, national and regional plans, and programme design and evaluation. Often external funds support such surveys.

Generally, the response rate of such surveys in rural areas is very high, particularly if the purpose of the survey is well understood and the confidentiality of the data respected. The reluctance of the disadvantaged, for example those living in shanty towns, to co-operate is easily appreciated. A sensitive approach that will encourage their interest and co-operation in the survey is essential. If areas are frequently surveyed without any follow-up action, or if government agents are suspected of collecting information for tax purposes, response rates are likely to be low. Bias can be introduced if people think that by reporting very low intakes, they will receive food, financial, or other aid from the survey agency.

In many developing countries, the majority of people live in rural areas. The time required for travel between households and villages is an important factor to consider in the overall planning of the survey and in the scheduling of the survey teams. The logistical points raised earlier in this chapter are particularly important in surveys in the rural areas of developing countries.

12.4.1. Quantifying food consumption

The agricultural based economies of most third world countries are particularly evident in the food consumption patterns in rural areas. A large proportion of food is home-produced, some is gathered, and the remainder purchased. Food is seldom subjected to careful weighing or packaging. Thus, if quantitative information is required, measuring or weighing of food is the recommended method of data collection. While rural people in the developing world may have little appreciation of national or international units of weight or volume, they can be very accurate in their use of local ones (7.1.2). Amounts are often expressed in terms of bundles or the non-standardized containers used at local markets (empty bottles, tin cans, plastic containers, or such). This expertise can be used to advantage in a survey, allowing respondents to refer to locally recognized units or containers which the surveyor then re-measures in standardized containers. The number of containers used in any one household or village is likely to be small, so that once a factor of conversion is established, it can be recorded each time a specific container is used to describe volume. A measuring tape can be used to determine the size of units of food such as sweet potatoes, sugar cane, fresh maize cobs (corn-on-the-cob). In addition to the weight or measure, the information recorded should include the source of each food, whether it was raw or cooked, and how it was cooked, so that the proper codes for composition and waste are used.

12.4.2. Seasonal considerations

The season of the year is a very strong influence on rural life. This has several implications for food consumption surveys. The seasonal nature of the food supply is particularly important. In post-harvest and dry seasons, food consumption can be remarkably different in quantity, variety, and quality from before-harvest and wet season intakes. The seasonal availability of fruits, vegetables, berries, and other gathered foods increases the consumption of specific nutrients that may be in very poor supply during other seasons. This variability may be particularly important in the food consumption of children who frequently take snacks of gathered foods. Food consumption surveys in the rural areas need to be carefully timed so that they intentionally measure food consumption during the two or three main seasons of hunger or plenty. Otherwise, they may be planned to capture a more-or-less average consumption during a carefully chosen neutral season. Work patterns of agricultural and rural life are also influenced by season. Survey visits should be planned to avoid times of peak labour demands, particularly those of women, and be scheduled for the convenience of the household. Because of the likely higher consumption of food on market day or the day following, surveys should be organized so that these days are not over represented. If food frequencies are sought, it may be easier for survey subjects to describe them in relation to agricultural or local events calendars rather than in the terms of days, weeks or months commonly used in urban areas. The logistics of travel are also influenced by season. The accessability of roads, bridges, and rivers may be an important seasonal consideration in scheduling a survey.

12.4.3. Local food habits, customs, and languages

A team of fieldworkers who are not from the local region need to be informed about, and be sensitive to the variety of local customs and practices they will meet. An awareness of religious, tribal, and local food practices is essential. Fieldworkers must show respect for local customs, courtesies, and language, and for local food taboos and rules relating to fasting and abstinence. Problems of poverty, local scarcity of water, fuel, and food need to be treated with sensitivity. The fieldworkers will need to make themselves familiar with local foods, food preparation techniques, and food patterns. They must be prepared to assign new codes and new descriptions to food composition tables when previously unknown foods are reported. They should also be aware of the reluctance of people to report the consumption of low status foods during periods of poverty or scarcity. The reader is referred to Chapter 7.2 for further discussion of the obervation and measurement of food consumption.

The common practice, in many cultures, of all family members eating from the same pot or plate, is an important consideration in choosing a survey method. In some households, the practice may indeed be dictated by the fact that they can afford only one fire, one pot, one food. Where food is eaten from one pot, household food consumption is much easier to measure than an individual's consumption. The fieldworkers should then pay particular attention to the pattern of food distribution in the household. In male dominated cultures, women and children may not receive a fair share of the foods prepared. Infant and child feeding practices are important to note in all such surveys. The composition of households in some cultures makes the determination of 'family' or 'eating' units difficult. In families consisting of more than one household unit, there may be a sharing of food which places special demands on the fieldworker recording the consumption of one particular unit. Meal frequency and the time of eating may not be as rigidly followed in some areas as in others. The frequency of meals may vary, particularly in areas where agricultural work and the distance to fuel and water are dictated by season. The time required to collect fuel and water are important variables to measure in food consumption surveys in developing countries. The monotonous nature of diets consumed in most areas of the third world may permit a good representation of food consumption in a shorter survey period.

Local languages and dialects abound in the rural areas of the developing world. In most cases it is not possible to organize survey teams that can work equally well in all languages, although it is useful to look for people who speak several local languages. Usually provision has to be made to hire and train local people as interpreters. It is recommended to keep the number of interpreters to a minimum because, unintentionally, they can be a source of error and bias. The problems associated with illiteracy, local languages, and dialects make it impossible to use written instructions or ask subjects to keep written records or diaries in such surveys. Colourful posters using pictures to depict the purpose and nature of the survey can be useful communication tools.

References

1. Emmons, L. and Hayes, M. (1973). Accuracy of 24-hr recalls of young children. *J. Am. Diet Assoc.* **62**, 409–15.
2. Sellitz, C., Wrightsman, L. S., and Cook, S. W. (1976). *Research methods in social relations* (3rd edition) pp. 531–3. Holt, Rhinehart and Winston, New York.
3. Statistical Office, Department of International Economic and Social Affairs (1984). *Studies in methods series F, no. 31: Handbook of household surveys.* (Revised edition) p. 21. United Nations, New York.

13

Economic appraisal of various study designs and methods

ALISON E. BLACK

13.1. The monetary costs of a dietary survey

There are five areas of cost involved in all dietary surveys. Two others may be involved with some studies. These are:

1. Personnel.
2. Equipment.
3. Transport.
4. Accommodation.
5. Computing.

   For some studies:

6. Subjects.
7. Food analyses.

13.1.1. Personnel

Dietary surveys are expensive in terms of time and people. The main purpose of this chapter is to identify some of the factors that influence the labour costs of a dietary survey. It also gives guidance on the number of fieldworkers needed to obtain a given number of records in a given time or, conversely, on how many collected records it would be reasonable to expect from a given number of workers in a given time.

13.1.2. Equipment

This includes dietary scales, food models, replicas, standard utensils, books or forms for recording food intake, and general stationery supplies (see also 8.1).

Equipment is the least of the expenses of a dietary survey and should not be regarded as an area for economy. If for example, the number of scales is inadequate there can be delays and frustrations among the field-workers.

13.1.3. Transport

The specific costs of transport will depend on the geographical area to be covered and local conditions. They can be nil if the fieldworkers live in the area under study and walk to their assignments. They can be considerable if it is necessary to supply, maintain, and fuel vehicles suitable for covering rough terrain in isolated areas. Travel also costs time. This should be taken into account when assessing the number of fieldworkers needed.

13.1.4. Accommodation

When fieldworkers live in and work from their own homes, costs of accommodation are nil.

If a survey is conducted in a number of different towns, then fieldworkers are likely to move around and require accommodation in hotels for some or all of the time.

If a survey is conducted in a remote and primitive area it may be necessary to provide everything. This would include shelter in the form of tents, locally built huts, or houses, all foods, and also domestic supplies.

13.1.5. Computing

Nowadays, dietary surveys are rarely completed without the use of computing facilities to calculate nutrient intakes and to handle the statistical analysis of results. Calculations for a small study of clinical patients can probably be accommodated on a desk-top microcomputer. However, the volume of data collected from a large scale survey will require access to a mini- or main-frame computer.

Computing costs may include:

1. Hardware costs: either buying a computer and perhaps also employing the expertise to run it, or buying time on someone else's computer.

2. Database costs: food composition tables must be available in a readable form for the computer. National food tables may already be purchaseable on magnetic tape or computer disk. If not, someone must be employed to compile the database to be used.

3. Software costs: either the purchase of a suitable program to calculate nutrient intakes or the employment of a programmer to develop a specific program for the survey. Statistical packages may be needed to examine the data.

4. Operating and maintenance costs: someone will be required to enter the raw data from the dietary records on to file in the computer. This

needs to be budgeted either in terms of the workload for the nutritionists and therefore in the labour costs of the survey, or for another individual. In addition, databases need updating by adding new items to food composition files and nutrient analysis programs require modification as the team discovers that results require to be calculated in new ways.

13.2. Costs in terms of respondent burden

13.2.1. Postal questionnaire

This method is suitable only when using carefully designed questionnaires that require precise and simple answers from the respondents. Respondent burden is minimal—only the time taken to complete the form.

13.2.2. Retrospective methods (24-hour recall, dietary history)

All retrospective methods place minimal burden on the respondent, since the assessment can only be done by interview. A 24-hour recall may take 15 to 30 minutes or a dietary history 60 to 90 minutes. Taking longer than 90 minutes is probably unproductive, as it is tiring for both respondent and interviewer. The respondent burden is slightly greater when repeated 24-hour recalls are needed.

13.2.3. Prospective studies in literate communities

In literate communities, it is normal to ask respondents to keep the records themselves. This places a considerable burden on them.

13.2.4. Precise weighing method

The respondent might be asked to weigh ingredients separately, combined, and during meal preparation, before and after cooking, and when served, before consumption. This is a great burden and only possible in studies with small numbers of highly motivated volunteers.

13.2.5. Weighed inventory method

The respondent weighs and records all food and meals as served. This demands a high degree of cooperation. In communities accustomed to using kitchen scales cooperation can be satisfactorily maintained. It is not as easy to do so in communities using standard cups or other utensils for cooking measures. Cooperation rates of 60 to 85 per cent can be achieved, but they become less as the educational level of the respondent declines.

13.2.6. Estimated records

Although the burden on the respondent is less when foods are recorded in household measures, this method still requires good cooperation. First, the respondent must remember to write everything down; second, a mental effort must be made to decide what 'measure' has been eaten; third, there may be a relatively long interview, when the fieldworker collects the record after checking it through with the respondent, to obtain more precise descriptions of foods and their quantities. However, better cooperation can be maintained with this method rather than the weighed inventory, particularly among the less well-educated.

13.2.7. Prospective studies in illiterate communities

In these circumstances it is the fieldworker who keeps the written records. However, the cooperation of subjects is essential at all meal times to enable the fieldworker to weigh foods and containers. The respondent's burden can therefore be considerable in terms of interference with the pattern of daily life and the invasion of privacy.

13.3.　Maintaining co-operation of respondent

Generally, the desirable length of a diet record for scientific and statistical reasons (Chapters 6 and 10) is longer than is practicable in terms of cost or respondent burden. However, in highly motivated groups, records have been maintained over long periods of time. A group of dietitians kept weighed records every sixth day for a year,[1] and a group of mothers kept records at monthly intervals throughout pregnancy and the first year of their infants' life.[2]

The extent to which cooperation from respondents can be obtained and maintained is described in Chapter 14.

13.4.　Labour costs of food consumption surveys

13.4.1. Planning

In this context, the term 'fieldworker' applies to both qualified nutritionists/dietitians and their unqualified assistants. It is unusual for more than one, or at most three, qualified nutritionists to be employed. When larger numbers are employed, the assistants are usually local people. They are educated and literate, but not necessarily qualified in nutrition. These assistants will be trained and supervised by the nutritionist. The term 'nutritionist' and 'assistant' will be used where it is necessary to distinguish between them.

Tables 13.1, 13.2 and 13.3 (at end of chapter) summarize the main features of fourteen dietary surveys and attempt to quantify the workload involved in differing circumstances.

There is one major difference between weighed records from illiterate and literate communities. In the former the food records are kept by the fieldworkers who must, therefore, be present at all meal times. For this reason they can only supervise one respondent at a time, unless several live and eat together. In literate communities, it is usual for respondents to keep their own records. One fieldworker can then supervise several respondents at a time, since visits are not necessary at meal times.

Dietary surveys can be considered as having four stages: initial high level planning, field planning, collecting and processing dietary records, and data analysis and writing the report.

Initial high level planning
This includes designing the study, acquiring funding and obtaining permissions from the highest levels of interested bodies such as Ministers of Health, local government authorities, and/or hospital ethical committees (Chapters 7 and 14). This is usually the concern of the project leader and can be a very long process. Fieldworkers are unlikely to be involved at this stage. They are not usually employed until funding is available.

Field planning
This includes getting things organized, preparing the way with village headmen, hospital consultants, school heads, or anyone else whose territory will be used, designing forms, buying equipment, practising techniques, testing questionnaires etc. The fieldworker is very involved at this stage.

Collecting and processing dietary records
Collecting is the main concern of the fieldworker and ends with tabulations of the calculated nutrient intakes, or whatever measure of dietary intake is being used.

Data analysis
To do this one studies the calculated nutrient intakes and relates them to the other variables examined, looks for answers to the questions originally asked, and applies statistical tests. The fieldworker may or may not be involved. A nutritionist/dietitian fieldworker may be

employed solely to obtain dietary records, code and compute them, then pass the data to the project leader for study, analysis, and report writing. An unqualified assistant may do no more than collect the diet records and pass them to the nutritionist for coding. A PhD student conducting his/her own project does everything him/herself.

When calculating the work load in Tables 13.1 and 13.2, time spent on high level planning and on data analysis has been excluded as far as possible. In Table 13.3, a distinction has been made, if possible, between the workload which includes time for field planning, collecting and processing diet records, and the workload which only collects diet records (that is the actual fieldwork).

13.4.2. Organization of time

Basically the time spent on a survey is divided into two parts for work in the field and in the office.

Fieldwork includes:

- practical planning;
- recruiting the subjects;
- collecting dietary records.

Office work includes:

- assigning a code number and weight to each food item in the diet record;
- any necessary transferring on to a form suitable for computer analysis;
- any experimental work to confirm coding decisions;
- calculating the nutrient intake manually or by computer.

In general, office work uses considerably more time than fieldwork. Indeed, the time spent on office work is not likely to be less than half of the total time. It can be a great deal more, particularly in developed communities eating a wide variety of foods and using complicated recipes and convenience foods (6.2.2).

When rates of literacy are low, more time is spent in the field because the subjects under study must be followed about by the fieldworker(s). Less time is spent on coding because of the limited selection of their foods.

13.4.3. Fieldwork

Recruitment

As in study 2 (Table 13.1), the people eligible may be identified and contacted initially by the school head or personnel officer in the school or place of work. The fieldworkers first contact is, then, with people who have already volunteered. However, recruitment can take a very long time, as shown in study 3. Subjects were to be a sub-sample identified within a random sample drawn from the electoral register. Initially, time was spent extracting names and addresses from the register and sending letters to all of them. Each household was then visited. Before contact was established a significant proportion required several visits. Those with the desired characteristics were then identified in a short screening interview. Of the 720 households contacted, 74 were eligible, and 63 were recruited for the study.

Interview time

This is the time spent with the subject. If the dietary assessment is retrospective, by recall or dietary history, then only one interview is required. It might last from 5 minutes to 2 hours depending on the period to be covered and the detail needed.

A minimum of two interviews is normally required in a prospective study for each dietary assessment in a literate community. The first is to give instructions and the second is to go through the completed records to obtain all the necessary information that the subject might not have provided. Depending on the techniques used and the subjects' level of education, one or more intermediate interviews may be needed to check on progress.

In cross-sectional studies, the initial and final interviews may be 30 minutes to 1 hour in length. Any intermediate interviews are likely to be shorter.

In longitudinal studies the essential part of each interview becomes less, each time it is repeated. This can reduce interviewing time for later records, as with the school children seen at school (study 2). However, in other circumstances 'friendly' time takes over (see study 1 and next paragraph).

'Friendly' time

This is the interviewing time that must be spent on matters other than those strictly related to the study itself. Being sociable, shows the interviewer to be friendly and interested in the person, and makes her/him want to help.

The time varies. It can be minimal, as in study 10, where people were seen on a 'production line'. Friendly time may be of limited importance with individuals seen only in hospital where, perhaps, the mind can be concentrated on the study to be made. In home interviews, the person is on his/her own ground and the interviewer is the intruder. Here friendly time can take up to one half of the interview time. With people living on their own with few activities, such as some of the retired and elderly, this part of the interview can take even more time.

In the longitudinal study 1, the prospect of a regular visit and a chat was a major reason for the mothers' continued cooperation. Visits were typically 30 minutes, but could be twice this, and the length of time increased rather than diminished as the study progressed.

Friendly time can assume more importance in rural communities where time moves slowly, in communities where the formalities of social intercourse are strictly observed, and where cooperation must be obtained from isolated communities with limited education or knowledge of the outside world, and to whom the purpose of the study is a mystery. When fieldworkers live alongside their subjects of study for extended periods (studies 11 and 12) good social contact and relationships are vital.

Travel time

This is the time spent by the fieldworker in travelling from subject to subject. It may be possible to ask the subject to do all the travelling as in study 14, where all interviews were conducted in one location. In a study done from a hospital department, the subjects may be defined by their condition, for example Crohn's disease in study 9, and be recruited and instructed at a routine clinic. They can then be asked (study 6) to return at a later date either having posted in their record or bringing it with them. Where interviews are concentrated in institutions, such as schools (study 2) or places of work, travel time can still be low. It can also be low if all the work is done in one village (study 11).

Travel can, however, take up a major part of fieldwork time. This happens if home visits must be made over a wide geographical area to a group of people who are unusual in the population. These people may be vegans or subjects with ileostomies (study 5). It also happens when many miles must be walked through the bush, jungle, or mountains.

Time can be used most economically in cross-sectional studies when fieldwork can be concentrated both in time and geographical location. In longitudinal studies when each dietary assessment must be conducted on a specified date, economical use of time is more difficult.

13.4.4. Office work

Coding

After the dietary records have been collected, they must be put into a form suitable for computing nutrient intake. An estimate of the actual weight consumed must be assigned to each food item mentioned, choosing the most representative code for the food (or combination of foods) from the food composition tables (Chapter 8).

If every food item has been weighed and if the food or food mixture eaten can be described by a single item already present in the food composition tables, this task is neither difficult nor particularly long. A 7-day 'western' record might be coded in as little as 1 hour.

If, however, the portions have been recorded in household measures, in terms of food models or in verbal descriptions, it takes much longer to interpret the information obtained and decide on an appropriate weight. A single retrospective dietary history based on one week's 'typical' food intake probably takes 3–4 hours to interpret and code. However, widely varying estimates of time per diet record have been given in the studies analysed in Tables 13.1 and 13.2.

Coding time is also much longer when cooked dishes* cannot be assigned to a single food code in the food composition tables and must first be broken down into the component ingredients (8.3.4). In study 1 a difficult 4-day record could take a whole day to code. It may be advisable to expand the food tables with values for additional, appropriate cooked dishes. This adds to back-up time (see next paragraph), but it simplifies coding. In study 10 the basic UK food tables were expanded to include typical dishes eaten by Asian immigrants.

Obviously, time for coding will vary with the number of days represented by each record. A 3-day record will take less time than a 7-day record.

Where food choice is limited and meals are simple, coding takes less time. In study 11 some 400–500 single-day records could be coded in two or three days by the two nutritionists (about 5 minutes per record). In study 14, the results of one interview took approximately 20 minutes to code.

Back-up work

In general, when planning surveys, the part most often forgotten is the work needed to obtain the information to interpret and code diet records. The work includes for example:

1. Deciding on recipes for dishes to be added to the food composition tables and calculating the nutrient content (8.3.4).

2. Corresponding with food manufacturers to obtain information on nutrient composition (8.3.3).

3. Cooking a wide range of meals, or parts of meals, and weighing appropriate household measures of them.

4. Systematically buying foods from the local market to determine the

*Dish=a meal or part of a meal/snack containing one or more ingredients. It may be eaten cooked or raw, hot or cold. Examples are meat, vegetable, or bean stew, dhal, risotto, omelette, fruit salad, apple pie, custard.

weight obtained per standard volumetric measure, or average weights of pieces of fruit or vegetables (6.2.2, Table 6.8).

5. Eating the same meals in the same restaurants as respondents in order to weigh portions served.

6. Buying, cooking, and dissecting convenience foods and meals to discover weights and decide how to code them.

7. Walking along supermarket shelves reading labels.

8. Sampling actual foods, as served in homes or institutions under survey, for later laboratory analysis.

9. Systematically studying the subject's recipes and cooking methods.

This work is very time consuming, and impossible to quantify, since it is carried on intermittently between other field and office work, often as part of the fieldworker's own household shopping and cooking. There is no doubt if food composition tables must be compiled or expanded, an enormous amount of time is involved. In study 10 it was estimated that as much time was spent on 'back-up' as on collecting records or coding. In study 6 the investigator considered that setting up this section of the database took the major part of work time.

Information is, of course, accumulated over time and further studies carried out in the same centre will subsequently need less back-up work. Before study 11 began, for example, analysis of the Gambian foods had been almost completed.

Computing and cross checking data

Although in a survey with limited numbers, calculations might be done by hand, these days the conversion of data on foods eaten to a calculated nutrient intake is usually done by computer. The fortunate investigators have access to computer staff who receive the coded records, punch the data into file, write, and run the necessary programmes, and send the final print-out back to the nutritionist. The less fortunate have to do some of their own computer work. This was so in studies 7 and 9 where computing took from 31 to 40 per cent of the total time spent on the study.

In any study, time will be spent in discussions with computer staff about how work is to be done and to sort out any problems. In study 6 much time was spent sorting out problems associated with putting food composition tables on file. The computing process can also have problems. The print-out may be nonsense and much time is spent in finding errors either in the computer program or in the raw data. One single coding error, for example, can turn all the survey's data from grams to ounces! Unexpected values must also be investigated. Is that high-energy intake genuine, or has a large portion of strawberries (No. 817) been coded as margarine (No. 187)? Tidying up data takes time.

13.4.5. Numbers of dietary assessments and work loads

Tables 13.1, 13.2, and 13.3 summarize some studies conducted under a variety of conditions. Most of these also included clinical, biochemical, and/or anthropometric assessments. If possible, only the workload of the dietary studies has been assessed. Where the collection of other measurements and questionnaires could not be separated out, this has been indicated. By comparing the circumstances of any proposed study with the circumstances of those summarized here, it may be possible to obtain some realistic guidance to help in planning for the number of records that can be collected and the staff needed.

In Tables 13.1 and 13.2, the workload carried by the fieldworkers is assessed. For full-time projects (in Table 13.1) the number of records that each fieldworker attempted to collect per week, averaged over the total time spent in field planning, collecting and processing dietary records has been calculated. This represents the maximum, reasonable workload and is the crucial figure needed in advance planning. The number of usable records achieved is lower and depends on the cooperation of the subjects and how many records are eventually rejected as inadequate. This figure has also been calculated.

For studies conducted part-time (in Table 13.2) the total number of hours worked for each record collected has been estimated. From this, it is possible to estimate either the total number of hours' work needed to collect x records, or the number of records that could be collected by a fieldworker working y hours per week on a grant lasting z weeks.

In Table 13.3, the workload has been calculated in terms of the total number of records collected, divided by the total number of fieldworker-weeks spent on the project. It includes the time of both the nutritionists and their assistants. The workload for the period of actual collection of diet records has also been calculated.

The number of records collected per fieldworker-week range widely. Generalization is difficult, but certain trends are evident.

The records of UK and African Studies have been analysed for the numbers of records collected per fieldworker per week, that is the rate of record collection.

UK studies (Table 13.1)

The highest record rates were reached in studies 9 and 10 with no recruiting time, because recruiting was not done by the dietitian, there was no travel, and the retrospective dietary assessment was a single interview. Studies 6, 7, and 8 also had no recruiting time and no travel, but used a method assessing current food intake. This increased interview time and decreased the record rates. The rate dropped markedly if home visiting was introduced. Study 5 had minimal recruiting time and a

Table 13.1. Summary of studies carried out in the UK, by full-time workers

Study	Outline	Recruiting	Geography	Computing by nutritionists	Back-up work	Records per fieldworker per week		
1	**Nutrition in pregnancy and lactation** (A. E. Black, S. J. Wiles) Full-time, longitudinal, from research unit. Mothers and babies studied at home. 4-day weighed records collected monthly during pregnancy and 12 months post delivery.	By nutritionists in clinic and at home	All lived in base town and villages	No	Shopping, cooking, food tables, additions	Record-sets attempted	2.6	
						Record-sets achieved	2.4	
2	**Diet and dental caries** (A. Hackett) Full-time, longitudinal, from university department. School children interviewed at school. 3-day records in household measures collected 5 times over 2 years. Children instructed in groups; records collected in 20 minute individual interviews.	By school	Schools area 20 miles from base, but time used very efficiently once in school	No	Development of food models	Records attempted	16.4	
						Records achieved	14.4	
3	**Distribution of food within families** (M. Nelson, P. A. Nettleton) Full-time, cross-sectional, from research unit. Whole families studied at home. 7-day semi-weighed family records. Stage 1–3:	By nutritionists at home	In one town. Work concentrated in local areas	No	Shopping, cooking, meal sampling, for analysis. Food tables		Stage 1–3	Stage 4
						Total screening interviews	—	8.2
						Family records attempted	0.4	0.7
						Family records achieved	0.3	0.6
						Individual records achieved	1.4	2.5

	Volunteers and Stage 4: Random sample from electoral register screened first then eligible families studied.				for school meals	
4	**Nutritional status of poor children** (M. Nelson) Full-time, cross-sectional, MSc Thesis work. Children aged 1–12 in poor families studied at home. 3-day records in household measures+anthropometry +questionnaires.	By knocking on doors and screening for eligible families	Work concentrated in poor neighbourhoods of London	Partly	Shopping	Total households screened 16.1 Household records attempted 1.75 Records achieved 1.3
5	**Comparison of methods of dietary assessment** (S. A. Bingham) Full-time, cross-sectional, from research unit. Ileostomists living at home were studied by diet history + 24-recall + postal questionnaire for comparison with earlier 7-day WI.	By letter, and telephone	Subjects lived scattered over an area 50 mile radius from base. Travel time considerable	No	Development of food models	Record sets attempted 2.2 (none rejected)
6	**Diet and ischaemic heart disease** (M. Thomson) Full-time, cross-sectional, from hospital clinic. 40 year old men, 7-day weighed record. Random sample from medical practitioner registers.	By letter	No travel. Subjects were instructed at the hospital and returned records by post	No. But a lot of time spent in setting up food tables	Shopping, cooking, extending food tables for fatty acids and cholesterol	Records attempted 2.0 Records achieved 1.8

Table 13.2. Summary of studies carried out in the UK, by part-time workers

Study	Outline	Recruiting	Geography	Computing by nutritionists	Back-up work	Hours worked for each diet record collected
	Trial of high-fibre diets for diabetics (C. L. Henry)					
7	Part-time, longitudinal from hospital. Diabetics in cross-over trial, kept 7×1-day records weighed/household measures over 6 weeks. Repeated after a break of 6 weeks.	By doctor at clinic	No travel. Subjects seen at hospital	Partly	Limited	Records attempted (none rejected) 8.1
	Trial of tablets *vs* insulin for diabetics (J. C. Heald)					
8	Part-time, longitudinal from hospital. Maturity-onset diabetics 7-day records in household measures/weighed, repeated 3 times over 15 months.	By doctor at clinic	No travel. Subjects seen at hospital	No	Limited	Records attempted 6.5

9	**Diet before illness in Crohn's disease** (P. M. Emmett) Part-time, cross-sectional from hospital. Patients with Crohn's disease and controls from fracture clinic. Habitual diet pre-illness assessed by diet history.	By doctor at clinic	No travel. Subjects seen at hospital	Partly	Limited	Records attempted (none rejected) 3.3
10	**Rickets, osteomalacia, and diet in UK Asians** (S. Warrington) Families interviewed at a central location. Adults seen at home or in hospital clinics. School children seen at school. 7-day recall.	Not by fieldworkers	Limited travel. Most subjects seen at a central location or in hospital	Partly	Cooking and preparing portions for use in interview. Extending food tables with Asian foods and recipes	Records attempted (calculated on the total number of individuals surveyed) 2.0

Table 13.3. Summary of studies in developing countries

Study	Outline of study	Staffing and travel	Notes	Workload
11	**Nutrition of pregnant and lactating mothers in a Gambian village** (A. M. Prentice, S. B. Roberts) Full-time, longitudinal, in field station of UK research unit. All mothers in one village studied throughout pregnancy and 18 months of lactation. 1-day weighed records every week for mother and baby.	2 nutritionists, 6–9 assistants. All lived permanently in the village	Nutritionists trained and supervised assistants, and did all coding. Assistants collected the dietary records. Coded records sent to UK for computing of nutrient intake. Some food samples collected for analysis in UK.	Fieldwork: 11.9 1-day records per assistant-week Overall: 9.3 1-day records per fieldworker-week
12	**Nutrition of mothers and pre-school children in rural Ghana** (F. Shizuka and colleagues) Full-time, cross-sectional, from a Ghanaian research unit. Random samples of mothers with one or more pre-school children. Village 1 studied in harvest season, Villages 1 and 2 studied in planting season. 3-day weighed records and anthropometry.	2 nutritionists, 6 assistants. Phase 1: assistants travelled to village weekly, collecting one set of 3-day records per week each. Phase 2: assistants stayed 3 weeks at a time, collecting two sets of 3-day records per week each	Nutritionists trained and supervised assistants and did the coding and computing. Assistants collected dietary records and anthropometry. Shopping and experimental cooking also done.	Fieldwork: Phase 1: Harvest season 1.1 3-day records per assistant week. Phase 2: Planting season 2.5 3-day records per assistant week Overall: 1.1 3-day records per fieldworker-week

13	**Seasonal changes in food production and nutritional status among Mali farmers** (M. Martin) Full-time, longitudinal, from UK university department. All households (of 2 to 46 persons) in two villages. Repeated monthly 24-hour recall of household consumption over 19-month period (76 weeks). Also anthropometry and other questionnaires.	1 nutritionist, 4 assistants. All lived in the villages for duration of survey	Nutritionists trained and supervised assistants and collected data. Back-up work in markets and homes to identify foods and quantify measures.	Fieldwork: 2.3 households studied per fieldworker-week Overall: (including employment of nutritionist in Mali and UK before and after fieldwork and training-time for assistants): 1.8 households per fieldworker-week
14	**Food and nutrition in the Kigeme area of Rwanda** (E. Dowler) Full-time, cross-sectional, from UK university department. Adult sample drawn from mothers/fathers bringing a child to a well-baby clinic. 24-hour recall of food intake, plus questionnaire on food sources, land and animal ownership, etc.	1 nutritionist, 1 assistant. No travel	Nutritionist trained assistant. Both conducted interviews.	Fieldwork: 8.75 interviews per fieldworker-week Overall: 4.4 interviews per fieldworker-week

single interview for retrospective assessment, but travel time was particularly high since the subjects were dispersed over an area of 50 miles radius.

The lowest rate was found in stages 1–3 of the Cambridge family study (study 3). These however covered the pilot stages of a new and complex method of dietary assessment[4] and an enormous amount of back-up work (see also list of publications analysed).

When the procedures for both fieldwork and processing the records were established as in stage 4 from study 3, the rate achieved was very much higher. The time to collect records from one family in this study was very similar to that needed to collect a 7-day weighed record from one individual. However, the time needed for processing one family's records was equivalent to that of four or five individuals. This is what determined the number of records that could be collected. The figures of 2.5 individual records achieved, comes close to figures in other studies.

A low rate was also found in study 4,[3] which represents work for a postgraduate thesis. It is unlikely that thesis projects can achieve high rates, since the individual concerned is usually working alone, often collecting a variety of records, and is probably inexperienced in fieldwork. Study 4 also involved a lengthy recruiting process and was carried out in a low socio-economic group where co-operation was low (see also list of publications analysed).

Differences in back-up work account for some apparently curious variation in rates. Studies 6, 7, and 8 are at first sight very similar: no recruiting, no travel, 7-day prospective records, and similar interviewing time. However, study 6 was primarily investigating fatty acid and cholesterol intakes, and an enormous amount of work was needed to sort out and extend this section of the food tables. Studies 7 and 8 needed much less back-up. The difference between these latter two, lies in the fact that the investigator in study 7 did her own computing. If computing time is deducted, the hours per record fall from 8.1 to 5.7, which approximates to the estimate of 5.2 hours per record in study 8.

The figures in Tables 13.1 and 13.2 are overall averages. However fieldwork load varies, being heaviest in the middle stages of a study. It is helpful to know how many subjects one worker can be expected to survey in periods of concentrated fieldwork. Perhaps some guidance can be obtained from the following examples.

In study 10, 186 Asians were seen in two weekends (4 days). They came to the hospital and were passed along a 'production line' from 4 clerks, to 2 doctors, to 2 phlebotomists, to 4 dietitians. The dietitians saw them as families and not as individuals. Thus the interviewing rate was 4 or 5 families per dietitian per day, equivalent to 12 individuals. This kind of arrangement clearly requires special organization and it is working under a pressure that cannot be maintained for long periods.

In study 3, several weeks of fieldwork only were followed by much longer periods of office work only. The number of families surveyed per week per fieldworker during periods of fieldwork only were 1.9, 2.9, and 5.2 in stages 1, 2, and 3. In stage 4 the fieldwork load was 27.4 screening visits plus 2.5 families surveyed per week. This latter level of fieldwork was maintained for 13 weeks; it was however both emotionally and physically exhausting.

In study 1, at a busy period of fieldwork, an average of 4.3 subjects were surveyed per week, with a maximum of 8 subjects. This was achieved in four mornings, the remaining morning and afternoons being spent in the office. At this level of fieldwork, however, coding fell behind.

African studies

As in the UK studies, widely varying numbers of records were collected. This variation in numbers of records is due, essentially, to the same reasons as have been described for the UK. As is shown in Table 13.3 one of these reasons is the relation of the investigator or fieldworker to the target group. For instance, do investigators live in the community as in study 11, are there possibilities for transport as in study 12, and what is the willingness of the subjects to co-operate?

Another reason is the method used in the study. In studies 13 and 14 interview methods were used. Study 14 involved single, relatively short interviews in a central location. In this study no serious attempt was made to quantify nutrient intake. Coding and analysis were in terms of foods eaten and frequencies of consumption, so the numbers of records per fieldworker per day were very high. The numbers in study 13 are lower, because the investigator wanted to quantify the nutrient intake. The households involved in the study were more complex and it was difficult to separate the dietary workload from the collection of other data.

When estimating dietary workload, other factors such as holidays, sickness, staff changes, and time spent in training has to be taken into account. These factors are likely to differ between studies.

13.4.6. General conclusions

The main influences on fieldwork time are the number and length of interviews needed, the extent to which the interviews can be concentrated in time and place, whether home visits are necessary, and how much travelling is involved.

The main influences on office time are the number of days collected for each record, the complexity of the dietary patterns, the amount of back-up work needed, and whether the nutritionist/dietitian has to personally compute the nutrient intakes from the raw data of quantities of foods consumed.

Acknowledgements

To all those colleagues who generously provided detailed information about the conduct of their own surveys.

References

1. Black, A. E., Ravenscroft, C., and Sims, A. J. (1984). The NACNE report: are the dietary goals realistic? Comparisons with the dietary patterns of dietitians. *Hum. Nutr. Appl. Nutr.* **38A**, 165–79.
2. Black, A. E., Wiles, S. J., and Paul, A. A. (1986). The nutrient intakes of pregnant and lactating mothers of good socio-economic status in Cambridge, UK: some implications for recommended daily allowances of minor nutrients. *Br. J. Nutr.* **56**, 59–72.
3. Nelson, M. and Naismith, D. J. (1979). The nutritional status of poor children in London. *J. Hum. Nutr.* **33**, 33–43.
4. Nelson, M. and Nettleton, P. A. (1980). Dietary survey methods. I. A. semi-weighed technique for measuring dietary intake within families. *J. Hum. Nutr.* **34**, 325–48.

Publications relating to the studies analysed

1. Whitehead, R. G., Paul, A. A., and Rowland, M. G. M. (1980). Lactation in Cambridge and in The Gambia. In: *Topics in Paediatrics. 2. Nutrition in Childhood.* (Wharton, B. A., ed.) pp. 22–3. Pitman Medical.
   Whitehead, R. G., Paul, A. A., Black, A. E., and Wiles, S. J. (1981). Recommended dietary amounts of energy for pregnancy and lactation in the United Kingdom. In: *Protein requirements of developing countries; evaluation of new data.* (Torun, B., Young, V. R., and Raud, W. M., eds) pp. 242–6. UNU Federal Nutritional Bulletin (Suppl. 5).
   Whitehead, R. G., Paul, A. A., Black, A. E., and Wiles, S. J. (1981). Recommended dietary energy intakes for the first six months of life. In: *Protein requirements of developing countries: evaluation of new data.* (Torun, B., Young, V. R., and Raud, W. M., eds) pp. 259–65. UNU Federal Nutritional Bulletin (Suppl. 5).
   Whitehead, R. G., Paul, A. A., and Cole, T. J. (1981). A critical analysis of measured food energy intakes during infancy and early childhood in comparison with current international recommendations. *J. Hum. Nutr.* **35**, 339–48.
   Black, A. E., Wiles, S. J., and Paul, A. A. (1986). The nutrient intakes of pregnant and lactating mothers of good socio-economic status in Cambridge,

UK: Some implications for recommended daily allowances of minor nutrients. *Br. J. Nutr.* **56**, 59–72.
2. Hackett, A. F., Rugg-Gunn, A. J., Appleton, D. R., Allinson, M., and Eastoe, J. E. (1984). Sugar-eating habits of 405 11 to 14-year-old English children. *Br. J. Nutr.* **51**, 347–56.
   Rugg-Gunn, A. J., Hackett, A. F., Appleton, D. R., and Moynihan, P. J. (1984). The dietary intake of added and natural sugars in 405 English adolescents. *Hum. Nutr. Appl. Nutr.* **40A**, 115–24.
   Rugg-Gunn, A. J., Hackett, A. F., Appleton, D. R., Jenkins, G. N., and Eastoe, J. E. (1984). Relationship between dietary habits and calories increment assessed over two years in 405 English adolescent school children. *Arch. Oral Biol.* **29**, 983–92.
   Hackett, A. F., Rugg-Gunn, A. J., Appleton, D. R., Eastoe, J. E., and Jenkins, G. N. (1984). A 2-year longitudinal nutritional survey of 405 Northumberland children initially aged 11.5 years. *Br. J. Nutr.* **51**, 67–75.
3. Nelson, M. and Nettleton, P. A. (1980). Dietary survey methods. 1. A semi-weighed technique for measuring dietary intake within families. *J. Hum. Nutr.* **34**, 325–48.
   Nettleton, P. A., Day, K. C., and Nelson, M. (1980). Dietary survey methods. 2. A comparison of nutrient intake within families, assessed by household measures and the semi-weighed method. *J. Hum. Nutr.* **34**, 349–54.
   Nelson, M., Dyson, P. A., and Paul, A. A. (1985). Family food purchases and home food consumption: comparison of nutrient contents. *Br. J. Nutr.* **54**, 373–87.
   Nelson, M. and Paul, A. A. (1983). The nutritive contribution of school dinners and other mid-day meals to the diets of school children. *Hum. Nutr. Appl. Nutr.* **37A**, 128–35.
   Nelson, M. (1985). Nutritional goals from COMA and NACNE: how can they be achieved? *Hum. Nutr. Appl. Nutr.* **39A**, 456–64.
4. Nelson, M. and Naismith, D. J. (1979). The nutritional status of poor children in London. *J. Hum. Nutr.* **33**, 33–43.
5. None at the time of writing.
6. Logan, R. L., Riemersma, R. A., Thomson, M., Oliver, M. F., *et al.* (1978). Risk factors for ischaemic heart disease in normal men aged 40. *Lancet* **1**, 949–55.
   Thomson, M., Logan, R. L., Sharman, M., Lockerbie, L., Riemersma, R. A., and Oliver, M. F. (1982). Dietary survey in 40 year old Edinburgh men. *Hum. Nutr. Appl. Nutr.* **36A**, 272–80.
   Thomson, M., Fulton, M., Wood, D. A., Brown, S., Elton, R. A., Birtwhistle, A., and Oliver, M. (1985). A comparison of the nutrient intake of some Scotsmen with dietary recommendations. *Hum. Nutr. Appl. Nutr.* **39A**, 443–55.
7. Manhire, A., Henry, C. L., Hartog, M., and Heaton, K. W. (1981). Unrefined carbohydrate and dietary fibre in treatment of diabetes mellitus. *J. Hum. Nutr.* **35**, 99–101.
   Henry, C. L., Heaton, K. W., Manhire, A., and Hartog, M. (1981). Diet and the diabetic: the fallacy of a controlled carbohydrate intake. *J. Hum. Nutr.* **35**, 102–5.

8. None at the time of writing.
9. Thornton, J. R., Emmett, P. M., and Heaton, K. W. (1979). Diet and Crohn's disease: characteristic of pre-illness diet. *Br. Med. J.* **2**, 762.
10. Stephens, W. P., Klimiuk, P. S., and Warrington, S. (1981). Preventing vitamin D deficiency in immigrants: is encouragement enough? *Lancet* **1**, 945.
    Stephens, P. S., Warrington, S., Taylor, J. L., Berry, J. L., and Mawer, E. B. (1982). Observations on the natural history of vitamin D deficiency among Asian immigrants. *Quart. J. Med. New Ser.* **51**, 171–88.
11. Prentice, A. M., Whitehead, R. G., Roberts, S. B., and Paul, A. A. (1981). Long-term energy balance in child-bearing Gambian women. A, *J. Clin. Nutr.* **34**, 2790–9.
    Prentice, A. M., Whitehead, R. G., Roberts, S. B., Paul, A. A., Watkinson, M., Prentice, A., and Watkinson, A. A. (1980). Dietary supplementation of Gambian nursing mothers and lactational performance. *Lancet* **2**, 886–8.
    Prentice, A. M., Whitehead, R. G., Watkinson, M., Lamb, W. H., and Cole, T. J. (1980). Prenatal dietary supplementation of African women and birth-weight. *Lancet* **1**, 489–92.
12. None at the time of writing.
13. Martin, M., Dowler, E., Hoinville, E., and Tompkins, A. (1985). Seasonal weight changes for some and not others in a rural community experiencing drought in Mali. XIII International Congress of Nutrition, Brighton, UK, 18–23 August 1985. Abstracts of original communications, p. 153.
14. None at the time of writing.

14

Practical implementation

INGRID H. E. RUTISHAUSER

Introduction

The purpose of this chapter is to provide guidelines on the practical implementation of studies concerned with the evaluation of dietary intakes. As far as possible the material is set out in the order in which the various questions that need to be resolved are best dealt with, by those responsible for the dietary study, from the initial planning stage through to the final reporting of results.

Figure 14.1, adapted from Rutishauser and Wahlqvist, shows the principal stages of this sequence in diagrammatic form[9] and also the order of presentation of the material in this chapter. Details of the various questions to be resolved at each stage in the process are given at the beginning of the relevant section.

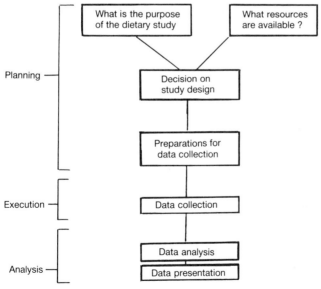

Fig. 14.1. The essential stages in planning, executing and reporting the results of a dietary study. (Adapted from Rutishauser and Wahlqvist.)[9]

As is evident from Fig. 14.1 the greater part of this chapter is devoted to the planning of dietary studies. This is because it is at this stage that the eventual success or failure of the study is determined. A study of the literature and practical information from persons with experience would make a good start. Inadequate planning leads to the collection not only of unrepresentative data but also data that is likely to be of poor quality. There is no point in analysing such data and therefore no point in carrying out a poorly planned study. Poorly planned dietary studies are a waste of scarce resources since data which is unrepresentative and inaccurate can be even more misleading than no data at all.

Data analysis and presentation are also highlighted because they are crucial to the final outcome of the study. If the study has no impact, was it worth doing? Making the results of dietary intake studies available in an intelligible and useful form not only to scientific journals but also to those agencies, both governmental and voluntary, which are responsible for the planning and allocation of food supplies, is clearly important. Sabry warns against the kind of scientific writing which reads more like a conversation between computers than a document with important practical implications for people.[10]

Adequate time and resources for data analysis and presentation need to be allowed for in the planning of dietary studies. If this is not done, analysis is limited because it must be completed before funds run out or it is greatly delayed because insufficient resources have been allocated to it. The final sections of this chapter are therefore devoted to a discussion of the requirements for effective data analysis and dissemination in dietary studies.

14.1. Deciding on a study design

What is the purpose of the study?
- Who is to be studied;
- what kind of information is required;
- what precision is required?

What resources are available?
- How much money;
- what kind of personnel;
- what equipment and facilities?

14.1.1. Step 1: Stating the purpose

In order to decide on a suitable study design and protocol the first essential is to know the purpose of the study; that is to state specifically

Table 14.1. Some examples of questions which might form the purpose of a dietary study

---

A. What is the role of snack foods in the diet of teenage girls?

B. Is there a difference in the level of energy intake between bus-drivers and bus-conductors?

C. Is sodium intake during pregnancy related to weight gain over this time?

D. What proportion of infants are solely breast-fed for at least 6 months?

---

the aims of the study. Table 14.1 lists some examples of specific study aims and these will be used to illustrate the basis for decisions about various aspects of study design (see also Chapters 4 and 6: Introduction).

The objectives of a study may be purely descriptive, as is the case of studies A and D, or the objective may be to compare the food intake, or diet, of two or more groups of individuals as in study B, or to study the relationships between dietary and physiological parameters as in study C.

The objectives of the study usually define both the group which is to be studied and the kind of dietary information which is required. For example in study A the group of interest is teenage girls while in study C it is bus-drivers and bus-conductors. In Chapter 6 (Introduction) four types of dietary information were identified. They all refer to quantitative data, although type 3 information can sometimes be obtained by using qualitative assessments. In Table 14.1 the examples A, B, and C ask for quantitative data and study D qualitative data.

The time frame of the study to be decided is: are current or retro-spective data needed?; at which time of the year and how many, and which days? Other aspects of the choice of a dietary protocol are not always so clear cut. For example in the case of study A, should the data be obtained by interview (retrospectively) or by recording (currently)? The answer to this question depends on two other criteria which the investigator needs to determine in the context of the study objectives:

1. How important is the representativeness of the sample?

2. How precisely is it necessary to determine dietary intake?

14.1.2. Step 2: The representativeness and an appropriate sampling frame

The study group needs to be representative, whenever it is intended to use the data obtained from the sample of individuals (or households) studied, to make inferences about the population from which they come. Generally this is the case, except in very special circumstances where the group being studied is the whole population (e.g. a whole village or the clients of a particular health centre). It is usually advisable, therefore, to ensure, as far as possible, the representativeness of the sample. The most common way of doing this is to select a random sample. A random sample gives all members of the population of interest an equal chance of being included in the sample. It requires a complete list of all the members of the population from which to select the sample, either by using a 'random number' table or a systematic approach such as selecting every tenth name on the list, the first of which is a random selection. Obtaining a complete list of the population is easier for some groups than others, for example, infants (birth records) and schoolchildren (school registers), and employed persons (employers' payroll). In some studies a general population listing may need to be used, such as electoral rolls, telephone listings, or household registers, and in others a sampling frame may actually have to be constructed by carrying out a population census. It is important to realize that some available lists are not complete. For example, a list of clinic attenders will inevitably exclude persons who do not attend the clinic in question, and lists, such as electoral rolls and telephone directories, usually are under-representative of some groups in the population such as migrants, non-ratepayers, young people, and those of lower socio-economic status.

In general methods which make the least demands on the subject — generally short-term interview methods — give the highest response rates and are, therefore, selected in preference to more demanding methods such as weighed or measured records. These may either not be feasible (lack of suitable equipment or inability of subjects to keep written records) or only acceptable to a limited proportion of the population of interest.

14.1.3. Step 3: The level of precision required and estimating the sample size

The level of precision required depends on the question being asked and determines the size of the study sample needed. The required level of precision is that which is adequate to provide a clear answer to the question(s) the study is intended to answer. For example, in a study designed to provide information on the average intake of a particular group, it is necessary to decide on the acceptable confidence interval for the mean (e.g. mean plus or minus 5, 10 or 20 per cent). Note that the magnitude of the confidence interval depends not only on the number of subjects included in the study but also on the variability in intake of the food or nutrient being studied. The greater the number of subjects, the smaller the confidence interval and the more precise the estimate of the population mean. The greater the variability, the greater the confidence interval and the less precise the estimate of the population mean for a

Table 14.2. 95 per cent confidence limits of sample mean expressed as percent deviation from population mean in relation to sample size and nutrient variability

Nutrient	Sample size					
	5	10	25	50	100	200
	Per cent deviation					
Energy	32	18	14	10	7	5
Cholesterol	53	31	24	17	12	8

Source: Beaton *et al.*[3]

given sample size. Table 14.2 illustrates the influence of both sample size and individual nutrient intake variability on the confidence limits for mean intake in a group.[3]

In a study intended to compare the nutrient intake levels of two groups, it is necessary to decide what level of difference between the groups is considered to be of practical significance. This is the basis for studying a sample large enough to enable detection of such a difference, if it exists, with an 80–90 per cent chance of success. The calculation of sample size is based on statistical information about the data. This is the variance and the level of significance and power required (chance of detecting a given difference if it exists), but the choice of the level of difference which is of practical significance is based on nutritional knowledge and experience. The investigator, not the statistician, decides what this difference should be. The statistician uses this information in conjunction with the statistical data on the variance of the parameter(s) in question to determine the appropriate sample size.

14.1.4. Step 4: The feasibility of the proposed survey

Once the required sample size is known it can then be decided whether the proposed study is possible or whether the desirable sample size is zero (i.e. the study should not be carried out). Essentially the question is: 'Are adequate resources available to carry out the proposed study?'. These resources include money, time, personnel, and the necessary equipment as well as computer and other facilities required to collect and process the data. It is not possible here to discuss in detail what is adequate, since this will vary from place-to-place, but it is important to emphasize that resources must be considered before an appropriate study design can be decided upon (Chapter 13).

Dietary information can be obtained in several different ways some of which may be much more cost-effective, either in terms of time or money, depending on the particular circumstances. It is clearly important to select the most cost-effective approach for a given situation, provided that it does not influence the purpose of the study.

In practice, the most appropriate and cost-effective study protocol is the one which provides just sufficient data to fulfil the study's aim. Collecting more data than is really needed to answer the question posed by the study is clearly neither cost-effective nor justifiable on scientific or ethical grounds.

14.2. Preparations for data collection

Having decided on a study design it is now necessary to prepare for the survey by designing survey forms, obtaining equipment, recruiting and training survey staff, and recruiting subjects. Finally, the survey procedures need to be tested, in a pilot study, on a small group similar to the study sample in order to find out about any practical problems before the actual study commences.

14.2.1. Step 1: Design and preparation of survey forms

Survey forms should be easy to complete, both for subjects and for investigators. In practice the form should: give clear instructions; have a logical lay-out; use a sequence in which information needs to be recorded either by subject or interviewer; provide adequate space for recording information; and leave enough space for direct coding of dietary and other relevant data suitable for computer entry. This avoids unnecessary transfer of information. Examples of various types of survey forms are provided in Fig. 14.2–14.4.

Figure 14.2 illustrates a simple form, suitable for the recording of dietary information by subjects in studies where weighed or measured records of intake are being kept. Forms of this type are best provided as a small (A5-format) booklet which is easy to carry around and also avoids repititious recording of basic data when more than one day's information is being recorded. The recording section of such a booklet needs to be preceded by clear instructions on what to weigh or measure, how to weigh or measure, and how to describe the foods which are recorded, in adequate detail for subsequent coding of the data.

Figure 14.3 illustrates the basic lay-out of a food frequency questionnaire. The purpose of such a questionnaire is to obtain a picture of the usual dietary intake over a period of time, in terms of the frequency of consumption of the foods eaten and the amount usually consumed. A problem can arise with this kind of questionnaire when a wide range of foods is available for consumption and consequently a large number of foods (more than 50) must be listed. This is to ensure that earlier and

DATE: ....   DAY OF WEEK: ....

| TIME | TYPE OF FOOD, DRINK, ETC. | DESCRIPTIVE MEASURE | AMOUNT(S) | | FOOD CODE | AMOUNT(S) EATEN |
			SERVED	LEFT		

Fig. 14.2. Basic form for a weighed or measured dietary record.

later questions are answered with equal care. When the data are to be used in relation to an individual it may be necessary to divide the questionnaire into two or three sections, which are completed at different times. For group data, however, it may be sufficient to randomize the order of presenting the questions to avoid bias. This can be done by collating the pages of the questionnaire (with the exception of the instructions page) in all possible sequences.

The quantitative aspects of such a questionnaire also need careful consideration since different subjects may have quite different concepts of what constitutes a slice of bread, a cup of rice, or a small, medium, or large portion of meat or fruit (7.1.2).

Figure 14.4 is an example of a 24-hour recall record form, presumably designed for completion by an interviewer since there are no instructions about quantifying the food intake data. The form allows relatively little space for adequate description of the food items consumed except by a trained person (6.6).

14.2.2. Step 2: Provision of necessary equipment: weighing scales, household measures, visual aids

The type of equipment required for carrying out dietary intake study obviously depends on the method being used, e.g. weighing, household measure, or interview.

FOOD	STANDARD SERVE SIZE	(1) Never/less than once per month	(2) Once per month	(3) Once per fort-night	(4) Once or twice a week	(5) Three to five times a week	(6) Once per day	(7) More than once per day	COMMENT COLUMN
Custard	1/2 cup					✓			
Lamb chop-grilled	2 chops				✓				3 at a time
Fresh plums	3 – 4	✓(o)				✓(s)			
Bread/toast	1 Medium slice							✓	5
Peas	1/3 cup					✓			
Ice cream	2 scoops		✓(c)				✓(H)		Small serve
Egg	1 Medium			✓2					

PLEASE NOTE

The person above has:

     – A standard serve of custard THREE TO FIVE TIMES A WEEK
     – 3 Lamb chops ONCE OR TWICE A WEEK
     – A standard serve of fresh plums once a day when they are in the height of their season (s) but only occasionally or never when out of the main season (o)
     – Five slices of bread and/or toast per day
     – A standard serve of peas THREE TO FIVE TIMES A WEEK
     – A smaller than average serve of ice cream, once a day, in hot weather (H) and once a month in cold weather (c)
     – Two eggs, once per fortnight

Please notice that you do not have to use the COMMENT COLUMN for every food: only if your serve size differs or if you eat the food more than once per day.

Fig. 14.3. An example of a food frequency questionnaire.
Source: Baghurst and Baghurst.[2]

Weighing scales

If the dietary intake study involves weighing, by the subjects themselves, it is important to provide scales which are easy to read, easy to use, have a suitable range for weights, and are portable (7.1.1). The number of scales required will depend on the number of subjects who can be studied at any one time, plus spares in the ratio of about 1 spare to 10 in use to cover breakages, losses, late returns, etc.

		Type and		Where	Office Use Only		
Time*	Food Items	Preparation**	Amount	Eaten***	Food Code	Amount	Code

Name: _____ Date: _____

Day of week of recall: _____

* A.M. Breakfast ** Fried, baked, boiled *** Home
  A.M. Snack   Toasted   Restaurant
  Midday Lunch   Whole wheat   Carried Lunch
  Afternoon Snack   Fresh, frozen, canned   School
  P.M. Supper   Creamed   Senior center
  Evening Snack   Child care center, etc.

Additional Questions:

  Was intake unusual in any way? Yes _____ No _____

  If yes, why (in what way)? _____

  _____

  _____

  Do you take vitamin or mineral supplements? Yes _____ No _____

  If yes, how many per day? _____ per week? _____

  If yes, what kind (give brand name if known)?

    Multivitamin _____

    Iron _____

    Ascorbic Acid _____

    Other (list) _____

Fig. 14.4. An example of a 24-hour recall record form.
Source: Black.[5]

Household measures

In a study in which information is to be estimated by means of household measures it is possible to choose between the provision of sets of standard measures or the use of existing local measures (7.1.2). The use of standard measures often has limitations. Therefore it may be more appropriate to use the local measures already available and regularly in use in the household (6.2.2). If a home visit is made in the course of the study, it is not difficult to calibrate the relevant measures if given access to water and a measuring cylinder or suitable scales. Many foods which are eaten do not lend themselves to description in terms of household measures, for example, irregularly shaped items such as meat or fish and many 'piece' items such as fruits or slices of bread which can vary considerably in both size and thickness. Provision of sheets of squared paper with 1 cm or other suitable size squares, provides a simple way of describing the size of such items. They can be drawn in outline, without the uncertainty that is attached to the use of terms such as large, medium, and small, or the arbitrary use of dimensions in the absence of actual measurement.

Visual aids

If the dietary information is being collected at an interview, it is necessary to decide on the kind of visual aids which will be used to help in quantifying the amounts of foods consumed (7.1.3). The possibilities include pictures, photographs, food models, household measures and utensils, and geometric shapes used individually or in combination. Table 14.4 (shown at the end of the chapter) provides a list of the visual aids used for 24-hour recall interviews in a national dietary survey of adults in Australia.[6] This list is included primarily as an indication of the variety of items which may be useful as visual aids and is not a definitive list. The items required for any particular situation need to be determined on the basis of local experience and dietary habits. When visual aids are used to quantify foods eaten, it should be recognized that individuals vary in their ability to use different visual aids to describe the same food portions. Estimates of individual food items can be subject to considerable error, for example differences of 20 to 50 per cent are not unusual. Over a number of foods, such as a day's intake, cumulative errors are generally less, because errors cancel each other in opposite directions. Nevertheless its overall error may still be 20 per cent or more in some individuals.[8]

14.2.3. Step 3: Recruitment of survey staff

Questions relating to the recruitment of survey staff are when, what kind, and how many? The size and nature of the study determine the number of staff required. Chapter 13 provides information on the time requirement for different tasks in dietary studies, which is helpful in deciding on the number of people required. Usually additional staff for dietary studies are recruited for the purpose of data collection and for data processing. The kind of staff required for data collection can range from highly trained specialist interviewers such as nutritionists and dietitians, to interviewers with no background in nutrition, but with adequate training in the use of questionnaires. It is also possible to use staff with no nutritional background to conduct 24-hour recalls provided that adequate training is given (7.2.3). However, for short-term studies, it is probably more cost-effective to employ persons with a background in nutrition or food science when the interview is largely unstructured and quantitative information on food intake is required. Recruitment of survey staff should take place in sufficient time to permit not only an adequate training period to the study but also to enable them to take part in the pilot of the survey procedures.

14.2.4. Step 4: Training of survey staff; data collection, checking, and coding

Adequate training needs to be provided in all the tasks to be performed by the survey staff. Data collection procedures usually receive priority, but training in data checking and coding procedures, and in public relations, is equally important if these functions are to be carried out by survey staff. Training should be carried out, whenever possible, by someone with an intimate knowledge of both the survey purpose and of the range of practical difficulties likely to be encountered in the field.

Data collection
Training programmes for staff assigned to data collection should include: methods for establishing rapport with subjects; importance of observer impartiality; instructions on the amount of detail required; interview techniques (if appropriate); methods for checking consistence in responses; and practical experience in data collection under survey conditions.

   Whenever possible all staff engaged to collect data should be trained together. When this is not possible steps should be taken to check the standardization of procedures in different centres (6.2.2).

Data checking and coding
Training in coding procedures is best based on a previously compiled manual which clearly specifies the procedures to be followed. Particular attention should be given to procedures for situations in which data could be coded in more than one way, for example:

(1) inadequate detail for specific coding;

(2) items not listed in the manual;

(3) conversion of non-standard amounts/unit;

(4) treatment of data outside the usual range.

   The coding manual will almost inevitably need to be added to or modified in the course of the study. A detailed record of the timing and nature of all additions and changes must be kept, in order to ensure that all records are eventually coded in the same way.

14.2.5. Step 5: Recruitment of subjects

The basis for deciding on an appropriate method for selecting study subjects has already been discussed in 14.1.1. The actual process of recruitment involves contacting the selected sample by mail, telephone, or home visit in order to explain the study and obtain consent for participation in the study. It is often advantageous, at the same time as study recruitment is taking place, to alert the media to the objectives of the study so that, when approached individually, study subjects are already aware of the nature of the study and the role that they will be expected to play. Since some subjects will not respond to a letter or will not be available at the time of the initial telephone contact or home visit, standard procedures need to be agreed for follow-up. This involves deciding on the number of repeat letters, telephone calls, or visits which will be made before a subject is regarded as unable to be contacted. In selecting the initial sample it is usual to build in an allowance for non-response, based on previous experience. Nevertheless, every effort should be made to obtain the maximum response rate by taking all possible steps to encourage participation. This could mean extending survey hours, carrying out survey procedures at home when necessary, obtaining employer or school cooperation when appropriate, and generally making it as easy as possible for individuals to participate.

14.2.6. Step 6: Piloting survey procedures

Most survey procedures benefit from a pilot study in order to sort out any problems which are not obvious except when used in practice. The kinds of problems which are frequently identified by pilot studies are:

(1) questions which are difficult to answer or lead to ambiguous responses;

(2) problems with the use of survey equipment such as weighing scales;

(3) the need for additional items such as visual aids;

(4) inadequate or inappropriately worded instructions to participants;

(5) insufficient time allowed for survey procedures;

(6) aspects of the study which are likely to reduce response rates.

As far as possible pilot studies should be conducted with subjects similar to those selected for participation in the study itself. Colleagues are useful subjects in the planning stages, but should not be used in pilot studies. A pilot study need not involve any more than, for instance, a day's trial-run of the survey procedures with a suitable group of subjects. The trial-run of procedures should be followed by the normal checking and coding procedures and a discussion of the problems encountered, together with the methods for dealing with them. If major problems arise, the trial-run may need to be repeated, but usually, if the study has been carefully planned, it is more a matter of minor changes than a major revision. The timing of a pilot study, should allow sufficient time to incorporate any changes that may be necessary in survey forms or procedures well before the scheduled start of the study itself.

14.3. Data collection

1. Liaison.
2. Provision of survey facilities.
3. Arrangement of appointments.
4. Arrangement of work schedules.
5. Supervision of data collection and checking.
6. Transfer and storage of survey records.

The amount of day-to-day organization required during the data collection period of a dietary study clearly varies with the size, geographical location, and time-frame of the study. The important role of those responsible for the day-to-day organization is to ensure the smooth flow of data collection and handling. The basic areas to organize are included in 14.3.1–14.3.6.

14.3.1. Area 1: Liaison between community and survey staff

This is an important component of all studies, but is essential in studies which require representative participation in order to fulfil their purpose. Liaison should begin well before the data collection period, preferably in the early planning stages of the study, but it needs to be maintained throughout the entire study period. Participation rates can often be improved by clear explanation of the study's purpose and its relevance to the community. Explanations are not only given to the group directly involved but also to people with authority in the community such as religious, political, and cultural leaders. Those responsible for liaison also need to make sure that there is a mechanism for a quick response to day-to-day queries about the study, both from the general public and from participants. In surveys in which the participants themselves are primarily responsible for the collection of dietary data, regular support is necessary to maintain their motivation. Finally, liaison should also ensure good relations between survey staff and survey organizers. This is best achieved by making sure that organizers appreciate, and give enough credit for, the vital role played by fieldworkers in the conduct of studies. They should pay due attention to the practical problems encountered and reported by fieldworkers in the course of data collection.

14.3.2. Area 2: Provision of survey facilities

In addition to the recruitment of survey staff the data collection period requires the availability of a survey base or headquarters, adequate supplies in the form of stationery and equipment, and, in some cases, accommodation and transport for survey staff. The survey headquarters may be in a fixed location or mobile, but a central point of contact for participants and survey staff is always essential. Arrangements for the survey headquarters and for the supply of all the necessary provisions need to be made well in advance of the data collection period.

14.3.3. Area 3: Arrangement of appointments

In order to ensure efficient use of the time of survey personnel and to reduce participants' waiting time to a minimum, some kind of appointment system is usually essential. Although a relatively simple approach is to invite groups of subjects to attend, defined according to geographical, age, alphabetic, or other criteria, in most situations individual appointments are more appropriate. If the latter approach is used, it is more efficient to give definite appointment times and only make special arrangements for those unable to attend at the given time. Appointment schedules should be realistic and allow adequate time for all subjects to provide the necessary information without haste. The quality of data is much more important than the number of subjects seen per hour. The number of subjects can usually be increased, if necessary, but the quality of data cannot be improved retrospectively. If home visits are involved the visiting schedule needs to make adequate allowances for what is referred to as 'friendly time'[4] as well as for data collection and travelling time (13.4.3).

14.3.4. Area 4: Arrangement of work schedules

The arrangement of staff work schedules clearly goes along with the arrangement of appointments. However, since data collection may take less time than the subsequent checking and coding procedures, it is important to remember the relative time requirements of both procedures so that a backlog of data and records is not allowed to build up. If the survey takes place over a relatively short period of time, for example, over 1 or 2 weeks, the staff's daily workload can be heavier than in long-term studies. Nevertheless, in the latter situation, adequate provision needs to be made for staff recreation in order to ensure the maintenance of high quality data collection throughout the study period.

In arranging work schedules it is always safe to assume that under survey conditions all tasks are likely to take more, rather than less time.

14.3.5. Area 5: Supervision of data collection and checking

Day-to-day supervision of the data collection period has a number of aspects. These include:

1. Maintenance, as far as possible, of the planned schedules of interviews, visits, etc. within the limitations imposed by unpredictable factors such as staff illness, loss of supplies, failure of communications, or transport problems.

2. Maintenance of some form of quality control of the data collection procedures. This can be achieved by regular observation of data collection by trained staff or by the introduction, at intervals, of known samples or check interviews into the survey programme.

3. Ensuring that the data are checked and coded, where appropriate, as soon as possible after collection. The details of this process are discussed in 14.4.

The purpose of day-to-day supervision is to make sure, by regular review of a sample of records, that the process is proceeding according to the prescribed procedures set out in the coding manual. If there is a significant amount of inadequate or ambiguous information in records, the reasons for this must be established and eliminated, if possible, at the earliest opportunity.

14.3.6. Area 6: Transfer and storage of survey records

The final process in the data collection period is the transfer of the records or data to a central location for analysis. If the original survey records are to be physically transported by mail or public transport it may be advisable, depending on the circumstances, to use survey forms which enable duplicate copies to be kept at source, in case of loss. In any case it can be valuable for copies of the original records to remain at the survey site for use by local community workers. With the coming of modern technology such as facsimile and other forms of electronic data transfer, in many studies it will no longer be necessary for the original records to be physically transported to a central location. However, even if this is the situation, it is still necessary for all the original data—not only the coded or abstracted information—to be transferred in this way. During data analysis, questions often arise and cannot be answered except by reference to the original data.

Finally, whenever possible, the original survey records should be stored in such a way that they are accessible to, and readily interpretable by other research workers at a later date.

14.4. Data analysis

1. Checking dietary records.
2. Coding dietary records.
3. Computerized or manual processing of data.
4. Preliminary data exploration.
5. Statistical analysis.

14.4.1. Step 1: Checking dietary records

The process of data analysis begins with the careful checking of the information recorded on survey forms. This can only be done by experienced personnel who can distinguish between consistent and inconsistent information, between likely and unlikely amounts, and between adequate and inadequate description of the foods eaten. This process must be carried out as soon as possible after the data are collected in order that any necessary supplementary information can be found without further delay. Computer verification of data cannot be used for this purpose. It is intended only to prevent incorrect transfer and entry of data or to identify numerical data outside expected limits. Preliminary checking of dietary data requires trained personnel.

14.4.2. Step 2: Coding dietary records

Conversion to nutrient data (Chapter 8)

In many studies food intake data needs to be converted to nutrient data. The method by which this is to be done will have been decided upon in the planning stage (i.e. direct analysis or use of food composition tables or a combination of both). In the great majority of studies conversion from foods to nutrients will be by means of tables of food composition. When a comprehensive local table exists there will be relatively few problems in coding the data, provided that the foods eaten have been adequately described. However, in many situations it is likely that there will be at least some items for which local data are not available. INFOODS[7] has compiled a worldwide directory of food composition tables and this may be helpful in selecting an appropriate alternative source of food composition data. For commonly prepared food mixtures or meals, representative data on nutrient composition can be compiled on the basis of recipe ingredients and local cooking procedures (8.3.4). For specific food items, not available in local tables, choice of an appropriate value should be based on an alternative food of, as far as possible, a similar species, anatomical part, maturity, age, and method of preparation. When analytical data from more than one table of food composition need to be combined for a single food, for instance, macronutrients from one table and minerals and vitamins from another, it is essential that the data used are standardized to the appropriate level of moisture content, since this clearly affects the level of nutrient content. In industrialized countries, with a very extensive range of processed foods available for consumption, supplementary information will generally have to be requested from food manufacturers (8.3.5). Ingredients and recipes used frequently vary with the availability and cost of raw materials. This is particularly relevant to studies in which the fatty acid content of the diet is of interest. Investigators also need to remember that the preparation and processing of food can have important effects, not only on the presence and availability of vitamins and minerals but also on the nature of the macronutrient constituents present, such as the conversion of *cis-* to *trans*-fatty acids, starch to resistant starch and hydrolysis of disaccharides to monosaccharides.

Conversion of descriptive measures to weight

Records obtained in terms of descriptive or household measures usually must be converted to estimates of weight. Unless individuals have used standard measures during the recording period, information on the actual volume of the measures used must be obtained and converted by use of appropriate density factors to estimates of weight (Table 6.8). Appropriate conversion factors, if not already available, should be obtained, whenever possible, during the course of the study, particularly for seasonal items which may not be readily available at any other time.

14.4.3. Step 3: Computer or manual processing of data

The decision as to whether to use computers or manual processing of data, depends both on the volume of data to be processed and on the access to suitable computer facilities (8.4). In general, however, nothing is gained from manual processing of dietary data when computer processing facilities are locally available. Manual processing of data is not only tedious and slow but also quite likely to lead to errors.

Micro-computer programs for analysing dietary data and carrying out basic statistical exploration of the data are becoming widely available and they have the advantage of enabling the investigators to maintain direct contact with the data during the initial stages of data processing.

14.4.4. Step 4: Preliminary data exploration

Preliminary treatment of data should consist of basic descriptive statistics such as the mean, median, standard deviation, range, and frequency plots of the data. It is at this stage that any obvious problems with the data are most readily identified. The maintenance of computer files (listings) of the basic data for each individual in the survey enables apparently incorrect values to be traced easily and corrected, if necessary, before further processing (9.1.5).

14.4.5. Step 5: Statistical analysis

The type of statistical analysis to be carried out will already have been determined by the study design because it is dependent on the question being asked and also influences the kind and amount of data needed. The exact procedures to be applied will depend on the distribution of the observed data. It is perhaps not generally appreciated that dietary data constitutes not one single variable, but a number of different variables which do not necessarily have the same underlying distributions.

   Certainly a number of dietary variables are not distributed normally, that is they do not show a bell-shaped or Gaussian curve, but are skewed to the right. Figure 14.5, taken from Rutishauser and Wahlqvist,[9] illustrates the difference between the intake distributions of protein and β-carotene intake in a sample of Australian university students.

   The existence of different intake distributions is one of the reasons why it is important to present not only the mean and standard deviation of dietary data but also centiles or frequency histograms. These show more clearly the nature of the distribution and enable appropriate decisions to be made about the need for transformation of the data prior to statistical testing (9.2). Statistical advice is generally required at this stage.

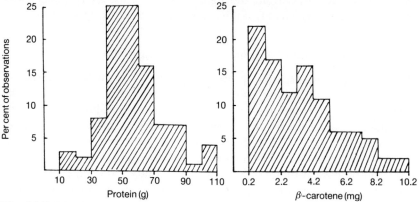

Fig. 14.5. Distribution of protein and β carotene intakes in Australian university students.

Source: Rutishauser and Wahlqvist.[9]

14.5. Data presentation

The way in which data are presented will depend to some extent on the purpose of the dietary study (i.e. whether it is basically a scientific enquiry, a description of the existing situation or an assessment of an intervention programme). The target to whom the information is of primary interest differs in each case and this needs to be taken into account by presenting the data in different ways.

14.5.1. Administration and planning

The majority of large-scale dietary surveys are undertaken for administrative and planning purposes. Examples of this kind of study are the British National Food Survey (NFS) and the American National Health and Nutrition Examination Surveys (HANES I and II). Results from studies of this kind therefore need to be presented, first and foremost, in a way in which they are useful to administrators and planners.

Questions that are of interest to these groups are the demographic, geographic, and seasonal distribution of food and nutrient adequacy. Data of this kind can be presented to advantage in ways other than the most commonly used tabular format, which is usually difficult to take in at a glance. Figure 14.6 is an example of an alternative presentation of

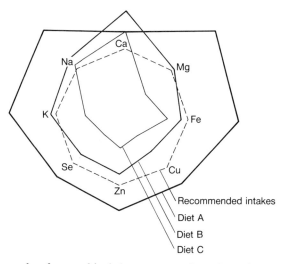

Fig. 14.6. Example of a graphical data presentation of nutrient comparisons of diets and recommended daily allowances (RDA).
Source: Varo.[12]

the nutrient composition of different diets which avoids the need to present extensive numerical data.

It is important that the information presented is both realistic and useful for decision making. Presentation of data which indicates only that the majority of the population have inadequate food intakes is not helpful for decisions about the allocation of scarce resources. Target groups for assistance or intervention need to be identified by appropriate analysis and presentation of the data. In this context simple comparison of intake levels with recommended dietary intakes or allowances (RDI/ RDA) is not helpful. Such a comparison inevitably overstates the real problem and other approaches should be used. Two such examples are comparison with an intake level which has significance in relation to the health status of individuals, such as the average physiological requirement, or a probability approach to estimate the proportion of the population likely to have usual intakes below their requirements. Table 14.3 compares the information provided by mean values, percentage of the population below the recommended daily allowances (RDA), and a probability analysis of the same data.[1]

It demonstrates the relative insensitivity of the mean as an indicator of the proportion of the population likely to have values below a given level of intake for different nutrients. It also illustrates the effect of using a probability approach in conjunction with the recommended daily intakes (RDI) to estimate the proportion of the population likely to have intakes below their requirements.

Table 14.3. Comparison of different approaches to dietary assessment of nutrient adequacy

Nutrient	Sex	Mean intake as percent of RDI	Proportion below RDA (percent)	Probability estimate of inadequacy (percent)
Protein	M	207	2	2
	F	174	13	2
Vitamin C	M	597	2	0
	F	437	5	3
Thiamine	M	137	31	14
	F	118	44	24
Riboflavin	M	195	9	4
	F	169	24	8
Iron	M	136	24	12
	F	79	84	20
Calcium	M	150	24	11
	F	147	34	21

Source: Anderson *et al.*[1]

More emphasis also needs to be given to the analysis of nutrient intake in relation to food intake. Usually food intake is converted to nutrient intake and presented as such. Much useful information is thereby lost. Planners have to provide food not nutrient supplies and it is, therefore, important to present dietary survey data in a way in which nutrient intake and food intake are related. For example, it is useful to present information on the major food sources of different nutrients for different groups. Examples include groups of different age and sex composition, ethnic or geographic origin, and level of nutrient intake. This kind of presentation of dietary data is illustrated in Fig. 14.7.[5]

14.5.2. Scientific publications

To a considerable extent the presentation of dietary data in scientific publications is governed by editorial policy and journal style. However, although it is usually necessary to present data in a concise, yet precise form which can be readily used by other investigators for comparative purposes (generally as numerical data in tabular form), nevertheless the primary objective should be the presentation of a readable and unambiguous report of the findings. It is particularly important that the reader should be able to distinguish clearly between the observed data and the author's interpretation of it. To enable the reader to do this the essential background information for evaluation and interpretation must be provided in the paper. This includes not only a clear description of the dietary methodology used but also details of sample selection, food composition, analytical methods, and statistical procedures used. Since only limited data can be presented because of space restrictions, it can often be helpful for the authors to make their basic data available, on request.

14.5.3. Education and intervention

Presentation of dietary data in a form suitable for educational purposes is particularly relevant in dietary studies where the findings have direct implications for nutrition programmes and policies at the community level. For example the finding, by a study, that regular consumption of a small quantity of dark, green leafy vegetables (DGLV) by pre-school children, is associated with a very low incidence of xerophthalmia clearly should result in a specific nutritional message for the community concerned. This message is unlikely to be transmitted to those for whom it is relevant if it is presented only as a scientific report. However, in the form of a poster or a regularly broadcast message about easily available varieties of dark, green leafy vegetables and appropriate out of season alternatives, or about how to use more dark, green leafy vegetables in

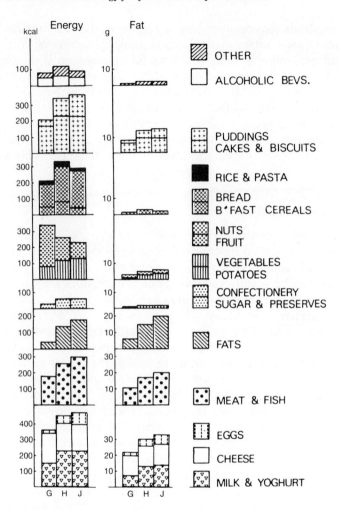

Fig. 14.7. Energy and fat intakes from different food groups in 36 dietitians, according to the percentage of energy in the diet derived from fat, G less than 36 ($n=20$) and J greater than 42 ($n=9$).
Source: Rutishauser and Wahlqvist.[9]

traditional dishes, it has a greater chance of reaching those to whom it is likely to be of benefit. Even though the investigators themselves are usually not in a position to undertake these kinds of activities, it is essentially their responsibility to ensure that those who are, such as community health workers and teachers, are provided with practical suggestions for the application of their findings at the community level.

14.5.4. Public media

The nature of media reports is brief and dramatic. In addition, most journalists and reporters are unlikely to be aware of the methodological limitations of a study. Consequently, reports of findings are frequently overstated in the eyes of those who are responsible for them. It can, therefore, be helpful if the authors themselves prepare short reports or statements for the media, particularly if the study findings are new, unexpected, or likely to have important implications for the group in question. Such reports will not only forestall inaccurate and over-dramatized media reports, they are also likely to be of value in improving community understanding of any problems identified and, therefore, community co-operation with measures designed to alleviate them.

References

1. Anderson, G. H., Peterson, R. D., and Beaton, G. H. (1982). Estimating nutrient deficiencies in a population from dietary records: the use of probability analyses. *Nutr. Res.* **2**, 409–15.
2. Baghurst, K. I. and Baghurst, P. A. The measurement of usual dietary intake in individuals and groups. *Trans Menzies Found.* **3**, 139–60.
3. Beaton, G. H., Milner, J., Carey, P., *et al.* (1979). Sources of variance in 24-hour dietary recall data: implications for nutrition study design and interpretation. *Am. J. Clin. Nutr.* **32**, 2546–59.
4. Black, A. E. (1982). The logistics of dietary surveys. *Hum. Nutr. Appl. Nutr.* **36A**, 85–94.
5. Black, A. E., Ravenscroft, C., and Sims, A. J. (1984). The NACNE report: are the dietary goals realistic. Comparisons with the dietary patterns of dietitians. *Hum. Nutr. Appl. Nutr.* **38A**, 165–79.
6. Commonwealth Department of Health. (1986). *National dietary survey of adults: 1983. No. 1. Foods consumed.* pp. 91–3. Australian Government Publishing Service, Canberra.
7. INFOODS. (1986). *International directory of food composition tables.* International Network of Food Data Systems Secretariat, Massachusetts Institute of Technology, Cambridge, USA.
8. Rutishauser, I. H. E. (1982). Food models, photographs or household measures? *Proc. Nutr. Soc. Aust.* **7**, 144.
9. Rutishauser, I. H. E. and Wahlqvist, M. L. W. (1984). The measurement of food and alcohol intake. *Trans. Menzies Found.* **7**, 97–110.
10. Sabry, Z. I. (1975). The cost of malnutrition in Canada. *Can. J. Publ. Hlth.* **66**, 291–3.
11. Simko, M. D., Cowell, C., and Gilbride, J. A. (1984). *Nutrition assessment.* Aspen Systems Corporation, Rockville, MD, USA.
12. Varo, P. (1985). Nutrient diagrams: a way to illustrate nutritional quality. *J. Nutr. Ed.* **17**, 39–40.

Table 14.4. List of visual aids used in dietary interviews[6]

Food models	
Pork chop, with bone	3.5 oz 98 g — 77 g of meat
Pork chop, lean and fat, no bone	2.3 oz 64 g
Pork chop, lean, no bone	1.7 oz 49 g
Ham slices, lean and fat — cold	3 oz 85 g
Ham roast	2 oz 57 g
Bacon slice — fried	10 g
Beef slice, lean — roast	3 oz 85 g
Beef pattie — grilled	3 oz 85 g
Hamburger — fried	3 oz 85 g
Beef cubes	3 × 1 oz each 85 g
Strip steak	14 oz 392 g
Meat loaf slice	3 oz 85 g
Beef liver — fried	2 oz 57 g
Beef stew with vegetables	1 cup
Veal cutlet, no bone	3 oz 85 g
Lamb chop — lean and fat, no bone	4 oz 112 g
Fish cutlet (square)	3 oz 85 g
Fish fillet	3 oz 85 g
Tuna, canned	$\frac{1}{4}$ cup 42 g
Prawns, boiled — 4 shrimp	1 oz 28 g
Chicken leg, with bone — fried	3 oz 85 g — 57 g of meat and skin
Chicken thigh, with bone — fried	3 oz 85 g — 67 g of meat and skin
Chicken breast, with bone — fried	3 oz 85 g — 73 g of meat and skin
Chicken wing, with bone fried	3 oz 85 g — 52 g of meat and skin
Chicken — sliced dark meat	1 oz 28 g
Chicken — sliced white meat	1 oz 28 g
Chicken — sliced dark meat	2 oz 57 g
Chicken — sliced white meat	2 oz 57 g
Apple sauce	$\frac{1}{2}$ cup
Beans, green	$\frac{1}{2}$ cup
Beans, baked — no pork	$\frac{1}{2}$ cup
Beetroot	$\frac{1}{2}$ cup
Broccoli	$\frac{1}{2}$ cup
Brussels sprouts	$\frac{1}{4}$ cup
Carrots — cooked	$\frac{1}{2}$ cup
Cauliflower — cooked	$\frac{1}{2}$ cup
Corn, with kernel — canned	$\frac{1}{2}$ cup
Peas — frozen	$\frac{1}{2}$ cup
Potato — backed in jacket — cooked weight	200 g
Potato — French fried chips	60 g
Potato — mashed	$\frac{1}{2}$ cup
Spinach — cooked	$\frac{1}{2}$ cup
Tomato — fresh	7.5 cm diameter
Tossed salad	$\frac{2}{3}$ – 1 cup
Vegetable soup	1 cup

Table 14.4. (*cont.*)

Cheddar cheese slice	1 oz 28 g
Cheddar cheese cubes	3 × 1 oz 85 g (28 g each)
Cottage cheese	$\frac{1}{4}$ cup 55 g
Cream cheese	3 ts 5 g
Cheddar cheese wedge	8 oz 229 g
Whipped cream	3 ts 8 g
Scone (biscuit)	2″ diameter 5 cm
Bread white slice	10.5 × 10.5 × 1.2 cm (approx.)
Bread wholewheat slice	10.5 × 10.5 × 1.2 cm (approx.)
Italian bread slice	1″ thick
Farina (semolina)	$\frac{1}{2}$ cup
Macaroni	$\frac{1}{2}$ cup
Oatmeal	$\frac{1}{2}$ cup
Spaghetti	$\frac{1}{2}$ cup
Egg noodles	$\frac{1}{2}$ cup
Shell noodles	$\frac{1}{2}$ cup
French dressing	3 ts
Mayonnaise	1 ts
Peanut butter	3 ts
Peanut butter, spread	6 ts
Peanuts	10 (whole)
Sheet cake with icing	7.5 × 7.5 cm
Jelly	$\frac{1}{2}$ cup
Pie — 2 crust apple	9″ diameter (23 cm diameter) $\frac{1}{7}$ of pie
Pie — 1 crust pumpkin custard	9″ diameter (23 cm diameter) $\frac{1}{7}$ of pie

Standard measures
2 measuring cups (250 mL)
2 sets measuring cups
*1 set (4) measuring spoons — $\frac{1}{2}$ ts — 2.5 mL
$\qquad\qquad\qquad\qquad\qquad$ 1 ts — 5 mL
$\qquad\qquad\qquad\qquad\qquad$ 1$\frac{1}{2}$ ts — 7.5 mL
$\qquad\qquad\qquad\qquad\qquad$ 3 ts — 15 mL
*1 set (4) measuring spoons — $\frac{1}{4}$ ts — 1.25 mL
$\qquad\qquad\qquad\qquad\qquad$ $\frac{1}{2}$ ts — 2.5 mL
$\qquad\qquad\qquad\qquad\qquad$ 1 ts — 5 mL
$\qquad\qquad\qquad\qquad\qquad$ 3 ts — 15 mL
*Note: A metric TB (20 mL) = 4 ts (5 mL)
2 rulers — marked in centimetres and inches
1 sct 3 cutters — 7.5, 6.5, 5.5 cm diameter
(ts = teaspoon; TB = tablespoon)

Table 14.4. (*cont.*)

Household measures
- 8 glasses (tumblers)—calibrated to standard in fourths of a cup and thirds
- 5 wine glasses—calibrated to standard in fourths of a cup and thirds
- 1 custard cup—calibrated to $\frac{1}{4}$ and $\frac{1}{2}$ cup
- 5 cups/mugs—marked to indicate volume
- 4 bowls (cereal, soup, stew, pudding)—marked in parts of a standard cup
- 2 plates—different sizes
- Spoons—1 ladle
  1 large serving spoon
  2 teaspoons
  1 soup spoon
  1 dessert spoon
  2 table serving spoons
- Baking pans—1 loaf pan
  1 pizza or pavlova pan—large
  1 pizza or pavlova pan—small
  1 pie pan—25 cm diameter
  1 pie pan—20.5 cm diameter
  1 pie pan—22.5 cm diameter
  1 pie pan—18 cm diameter
  2 × individual pie pan (tart)—9 cm diameter
  2 × cake pan—20 cm diameter
  1 cake pan—oblong

Surface area guides
Squares— 16 square cm (4.0 cm square)
  20 square cm (4.5 cm square)
  30 square cm (5.5 cm square)
  40 square cm (6.3 cm square)
  50 square cm (7.1 cm square)
  60 square cm (7.7 cm square)
  80 square cm (8.9 cm square)
  100 square cm (10.0 cm square)
Discs— 16 square cm (3.5 cm diameter)
  20 square cm (4.5 cm diameter)
  30 square cm (6.2 cm diameter)
  40 square cm (7.1 cm diameter)
  50 square cm (8.0 cm diameter)
  60 square cm (8.7 cm diameter)
  80 square cm (10.1 cm diameter)
  100 square cm (11.3 cm diameter)

Thickness indicator
15 leaves—each leaf 3 mm thick
10 leaves indicates 30 mm thickness (3 cm)
 6 leaves indicates 18 mm thickness (1.8 cm)

INDEX